D1643452

MALNOURISHED CHILDREN
IN THE
UNITED STATES

Robert J. Karp, MD, is Associate Professor of Clinical Pediatrics at the State University of New York Health Science Center in Brooklyn. He is the Medical Director of the Pediatric Resource Center, Kings County Hospital, Brooklyn, Lecturer, Institute of Human Nutrition, Columbia University, New York, and Associate Director of the New York/New Jersey Regional Center for Clinical Nutrition Education.

MALNOURISHED CHILDREN IN THE UNITED STATES

Caught in the Cycle of Poverty

Robert J. Karp, MD
Editor

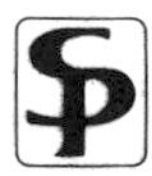

SPRINGER PUBLISHING COMPANY
NEW YORK

Springer Publishing Company, Inc.
536 Broadway
New York, NY 10012-3955

93 94 95 96 97 / 5 4 3 2 1

Library of Congress Cataloging-in-Publication Data

Malnourished children in the United States : caught in the cycle of poverty /
Robert Karp, editor.
p. cm.
Includes bibliographical references and index.
ISBN 0-8261-7330-6
1. Malnutrition in children—United States. 2. Poor children—United States—Nutrition. 3. Child development deviations—Nutritional aspects. I. Karp, Robert.
[DNLM: 1. Child Development. 2. Poverty—United States. 3. Child Nutritional Status—in infancy & childhood. WS 105.5.D3 M256 1993]
RJ399.M26M32 1993 362.1′989239′00973—dc20
DNLM/DLC
for Library of Congress

93-18736
CIP

Printed in the United States of America

Contents

Contributors

Steven Ajl, MD, is Assistant Professor of Pediatrics at the State University of New York Health Science Center in Brooklyn (SUNY–Brooklyn) and Director of the Breast-Feeding Clinic.

Ellis Arnstein, MD, is Medical Director of the Pediatric Resource Center Project of Albert Einstein School of Medicine, New York.

Andrea Berne, RN, was formerly with the Homeless Care Project of the Health and Hospital Corporation of New York City in cooperation with Beth Israel Hospital, NY.

Andrew Bostom, MD, is a graduate of SUNY–Brooklyn.

Rosalyn Bowser, RD, is a dietician at Brooklyn Hospital.

Joanne Bradley, PhD, EdD, is Dean of the College of Allied Health of SUNY–Brooklyn.

Linda Chabrier, MD, is a graduate of SUNY–Brooklyn.

Margaret Clark, MD, is Assistant Professor of Pediatrics at SUNY–Brooklyn.

Darwin Deen, Jr., MD, is Director of New York/New Jersey Regional Center for Clinical Nutrition and Assistant Professor of Family Practice, Albert Einstein College of Medicine, Bronx, NY.

Jeanette Fairorth, RN, EdD, is a school nurse at Olney High School in Philadelphia, PA.

Laurence Finberg, MD, is Professor and Chairman of the Department of Pediatrics at SUNY–Brooklyn. He is the immediate past Chairman of the Committee on Nutrition of the American Academy of Pediatrics.

M.R.C. Greenwood, PhD, is Dean and Professor of the College of Nutrition at the University of California at Davis.

Paul Harris, MD, is Associate Professor of Pediatrics at SUNY–Brooklyn.

Mary F. Healy, RD, is an Associate of the Camden Perinatal Project, Camden, NJ.

Mary L. Hediger, PhD, is an Associate of the Camden Perinatal Project, Camden, NJ.

Joan Hittleman, PhD, is Associate Professor of Psychiatry at SUNY–Brooklyn and Director of the Developmental Intervention Program.

Joanne Hurley, MS, RD, is Research Dietician at the Gila River (Pima) Reservation, Saccaton, Arizona.

Julie R. Ingelfinger, MD, is Director of the Pediatric Nephrology Section of Massachusetts General Hospital and Associate Professor of Pediatrics, Harvard University School of Medicine, Cambridge, MA.

M. Yvonne Jackson, PhD, RD, is Chief, Nutrition and Dietetics Section, U.S. Public Health Service, Indian Health Service.

Patricia R. Johnson, PhD, is Professor of Nutrition, University of California at Davis.

Francis E. Johnston, PhD, is Chairman of the Department of Graduate Anthropology of the University of Pennsylvania, Philadelphia.

Betsy Lozoff, MD, is Associate Professor of Pediatrics at Case Western Reserve University of Medicine, Cleveland, Ohio.

Borinquen Lugton, RD, is with the New York Department of Health.

Diane Markowitz, DMD, is Assistant Professor at the University of Pennsylvania School of Dental Medicine and an Associate of the Krogman Center for Anthropologic Studies.

Hermann Mendez, MD, is Associate Professor of Clinical Pediatrics at SUNY–Brooklyn.

Maudene Nelson, MS, RD, is Senior Dietician at the Institute of Human Nutrition, Columbia University, New York.

Marion Nestle, PhD, MPH, is Professor and Chair of the Department of Food and Hotel Management at New York University.

Renee Murray-Bachmann, MS, RD, is Director of Dietetics at St. Mary's Hospital, Brooklyn.

Denise Paone, RN, was with the Homeless Care Project of the Health and Hospital Corporation in cooperation with Beth Israel Hospital, New York.

Vivian D. Price, PhD, is Director of Program Development for Special Education for the School District of Philadelphia, PA.

Qutub Qazi, MD, PhD, is Professor of Pediatrics at SUNY–Brooklyn and Director of the Genetics Clinic.

Simon Rabinowitz, MD, PhD, is Chief of Gastroenterology and Nutrition and Assistant Professor of Pediatrics at SUNY–Brooklyn.

James Rempel, RN, MS, is Director of the Kings County Hospital Maternal-Child HIV Network, Brooklyn, NY.

David M. Rosen, PhD, JD, is Professor of Anthropology at Fairleigh Dickinson University, Teaneck, NJ.

Theresa O. Scholl, PhD, MPH, is Director of the Camden Perinatal Project and Associate Professor of Obstetrics and Gynecology at the University of Medicine and Dentistry of New Jersey–School of Osteopathic Medicine, Camden, NJ.

Trevor E. Sewell, PhD, is Dean of the College of Education of Temple University, Philadelphia, PA.

Carl Senft, MS, is a graduate of the Institute of Human Nutrition of Columbia University, New York.

Edith Snyder, MS, is a graduate student at the Institute of Human Nutrition, Columbia University, New York.

Peter Vasilenko III, PhD, was an Associate of the Camden Perinatal Project, Camden, NJ.

Theodore D. Wachs, PhD, is Professor of Psychology at Purdue University, West Lafayette, IN.

Stephen Wadowski, MD, is Assistant Professor of Clinical Pediatrics at SUNY–Brooklyn.

Myron Winick, MD, is Professor of Pediatrics, Emeritus, and of Pediatrics and Nutrition at Columbia University College of Physicians and Surgeons, New York.

Marilyn A. Winkleby, PhD, is Evaluation Director/Epidemiologist at The Stanford Five-City Project, Stanford University School of Medicine, Stanford, CA.

Patricia Giblin Wolman, EdD, RD, was senior WIC nutritionist for the State of Maine and is currently Professor of Human Nutrition at Winthrop College, Rock Hill, S.C.

Foreword

From a public health standpoint our course remains clear: Break the cycle of poverty by correcting the conditions leading to malnutrition and environmental deprivation. This may sound like an impossible task, but I can think of none that should have a higher priority. This book addresses this issue at the place where physicians and other health professionals often find themselves—in the gray area where judgment may take precedence over science, where public health policy and the relationship between mother and child are more important than clinical skills.

We have come almost full circle in the last 40 years in our understanding of the relationship of early malnutrition and subsequent mental development. In the 1940s and early 1950s, Stoch and Smythe (1963), after studying two groups of South African children, proposed that undernutrition early in life led to poor mental development. Herbert Birch and Joachim Cravioto, in a series of studies conducted mostly in Mexico, confirmed this view and extended it by proposing that the earlier the undernutrition, the severer the mental retardation (Birch & Gussow, 1970).

In the 1960s and early 1970s a series of observations begun by Kennedy, McCance, and Widdowsen, and extended by Winick and Rosso, and Dobbing and Sands concluded that early undernutrition permanently retarded brain growth by reducing the rate of cell division and resulting in a smaller brain with fewer cells as seen in many studies in animals as well as several in children (Dobbing, 1984; Winick & Rosso, 1969). It was tempting to conclude that the retarded mental development was caused by the permanent cellular changes induced by early undernutrition. The prevailing view was that severe undernutrition during the first year of life, often referred to as infantile marasmus, which occurred throughout the developing world and in poverty-strickened areas of the developed world, could by itself result in a brain that was physically and functionally permanently damaged (Cravioto, et al., 1966).

The social consequences were staggering. More than 300 million people throughout the world had suffered from severe undernutrition during early life. Cravioto and Birch suggested that early undernutrition set in motion a vicious cycle that led to retarded mental development, and reduced the chances of the child succeeding in school and the adult of acquiring the skills to move out of poverty. The result was a new generation fixed in poverty and susceptible to early undernutrition and a repetition of the cycle. A comprehensive review of these early concerns can be found in Birch and Gussow (1970).

In the early 1970s, a new series of findings added some complexity to the problem. Richard Barnes and David Levitsky described a series of experiments in animals that suggested that malnutrition alone may not have been responsible for the retarded development to which they and others had subscribed. Instead, they hypothesized, malnutrition accompanied by isolation from the normal neonatal environment may have been to blame. These observations suggested that in children the effect of the environment in which the undernutrition occurred might be as important or even more important than the undernutrition itself. Chavez suggested that early undernutrition led to extreme passivity in the child who demanded less and therefore, in a poor social environment, was even further neglected—another vicious cycle (Chavez & Martinez, 1979).

More recently, studies in children have begun to confirm this view. Children from middle-class families who had suffered severe malnutrition in infancy, such as children with cystic fibrosis, did not show any signs of mental retardation when examined 10 years later. Even children malnourished early in life in the poverty environment of the developing world showed marked improvement in mental development if adopted before they were 3 years old by middle-class American families (Winick, Meyer, & Harris, 1975). In the past few years the pendulum has been swinging back. Galler and colleagues (1984), in a series of studies conducted in Barbados, suggests that early malnutrition alone may indeed lead to subtle behavioral and neurological changes that persist. Most recently, Lucas et al. (1990) have shown that premature infants who are fed aggressively develop more normally than similar infants who are not as aggressively nourished.

What can we say today about the effects of early undernutrition on subsequent mental development? Certainly undernutrition per se permanently retards and distorts brain growth. Under the prevailing conditions within the Third World, early undernutrition, along with poor environmental conditions, can lead to permanent retarded development. Even when the environment is adequate, early undernutrition may have subtle deleterious consequences. Because even severe undernutrition in a good environment will result only in subtle behavioral changes, a less than perfect nutritional status may have to be accepted so that the child can survive. There are some basics, however. Young infants unable to consume adequate calories to sustain acceptable growth should be fed aggressively within the confines of safety.

MYRON WINICK, MD

REFERENCES

Birch, H. G., & Gussow, J. D. (1970). *Disadvantaged children: Health, nutrition and school failure*. New York: Harcourt Brace & World.

Chavez, A., & Martinez, C. (1979). Consequences of insufficient nutrition on child character and behavior. In D. A. Livitsky (Ed.), *Malnutrition, environment and behavior: New perspectives*. Ithaca, NY: Cornell University Press.

Cravioto, J., DeLicardie, E. R., & Birch, H. G. (1966). Nutrition growth and neurointegrative development and experimental and ecology study. *Pediatrics, 38*(Suppl.), 319–373.

Dobbing, J. (1984). Infant nutrition and later achievement. *Nutrition Reviews, 42*, 1–7.

Galler, J. R., Ramsey, F., & Solomono, G. (1984). The influence of early malnutrition on subsequent behavioral development: III. Learning disabilities as a sequel to malnutrition. *Pediatric Research, 18*, 309–313.

Lucas, A., Morley, R., Cole, T. J., et al. (1990). Early diet in preterm babies and developmental status at 18 months. *Lancet, 335*, 1477–81.

Stoch, M. B., & Smythe, P. M. (1963). Does undernutrition during infancy inhibit brain growth and subsequent intellectual development? *Archives of Disease in Childhood, 38*, 546–552.

Winick, M., Meyer, K. K., & Harris, R. C. (1975). Malnutrition and environmental enrichment by early adoption. *Science, 190*, 1173.

Winick, M., & Rosso, P. (1969). The effect of severe early malnutrition on the cellular growth of human brain. *Pediatric Research, 3*, 181–184.

Acknowledgments

In March 1989, several committees of the New York Academy of Medicine held a conference, "Nutrition, Children, and Health," with leaders of the pediatric and nutrition communities as conveners. The success of the conference in presenting the complexity of the relationship between malnutrition and poverty suggested to us that we could prepare a comprehensive text on the subject. Several of the presenters at that conference (Drs. Finberg, Ingelfinger, Lozoff, Winick, and Karp) contributed chapters to this book.

Several students at my own school, the State University of New York (SUNY)–Brooklyn, became involved early in the project. Individual thanks are given to them at the ends of chapters, but this is my chance to thank some other students who have worked with me in the past. Bill Haaz, Karen Starko, Jack Gorman, Nuchpakdee Mundhana, Edith Snider, Warren Matthews and Ed Decker are a few who deserve special mention. My faculty colleague, Annabelle Schaeffer, was a confidant when wise advice was needed. Two of our SUNY–Brooklyn pediatric residents, Francisco Sylvester and Luis Faverio, were extremely helpful in clarifying ideas. Carl Senft, as editorial assistant, prepared manuscripts for submittal to the publisher and provided thoughtful comments. Steve Wadowski constructed many of the figures. Special thanks to my colleague Swati Mehta and the entire staff of the Pediatric Resource Center (PRC) of Kings County Hospital. Pat Parker of the PRC of Kings County Hospital, Romas Srugas of Medical Illustration, several librarians, and Joel Stern at the Information Center of SUNY–Brooklyn were especially helpful. Victoria Rosen, PhD (for Part 1), and Maureen Gilmore, MD (for Section 3) provided exceptional guidance to me in the preparation of the final draft of the text. The support of the March of Dimes Foundation for my training in nutrition at New York Hospital/Cornell Medical Center from 1968 to 1970 is noted with great appreciation.

Most important for me was the support received from my family: first from my parents, Manny, Louise and Esther Karp, and from my wife, Linda Oppenheim who helped enormously in setting the dimensions of the text and in editing many of the chapters.

Malnourished Children in the United States was prepared under the auspices of the New York/New Jersey Regional Center for Clinical Nutrition Education, a project of the New York Academy of Medicine which was organized by Dr. Maurice Shils and is now directed by Dr. Darwin Deen. Questions and/or concerns are welcome. We invite comments from teachers who are planning to use the book in class or seminar setting. Please feel free to write to: The Regional Center for Clinical Nutrition Education, New York Academy of Medicine, 2 East 103rd Street, New York, NY 10029.

Introduction: A History and Overview of Malnourished Children in the United States

EARLY INVESTIGATIONS

Malnutrition is a complex disorder that has been studied for nearly 100 years by biochemists, anthropologists, dietitians, epidemiologists, and clinical physicians (Schneider, 1983). In 1913, Joseph Goldberger, MD, a physician trained in infectious disease, was sent by the U.S. Public Health Service to find the agent "causing" pellagra in the American South. Dr. Goldberger, known today as "the father of American nutrition," was able to discard the specifics of his own training and, instead, use principles of scientific investigation to identify the true cause: a dietary deficiency of the nutrient niacin. He observed that employees of hospitals or prisons in areas where pellagra was common never contracted the disease. "To this writer," Goldberger wrote in his journal, "the peculiar exemptions or immunity is inexplicable on the assumption that pellagra is communicable . . . the difference is in the diet of the two groups of residents" (Sebrell, 1955).

In his biographical essay on the life of Dr. Goldberger, W. H. Sebrell (1955) wrote, "[He] was well aware that pellagra was a problem of poverty and that only improvement in economic conditions would eradicate the disease. . . . [H]e could see the great economic and social advantages to be gained if the cycle could be broken and the disease prevented long enough for the stronger, healthier people to help themselves by improving their own food supply." Goldberger's studies alerted researchers to the importance of yet unidentified micronutrients present in the diet. This began the "biologic age" in nutrition research during which the connection was made between "a lack in the diet of 'special substances . . . which we will call vitamines' " (e.g., cholecalciferol (vitamin D) and rickets, ascorbic acid (vitamin C) and scurvy, thiamin (vitamin B_1) and beri-beri) (Schneider, 1983).

It is difficult, however, to determine how malnutrition was affecting children at that time. The contemporary literature is mostly descriptive, because the science of epidemiology was as primitive as the science of nutrition. As Holt, for example, noted in his 1911 edition of *The Diseases of Infancy and Childhood*, "In New York among dispensary and hospital patients, rickets is exceedingly common, and is seen chiefly in the foreign elements of the population . . . the greatest susceptibility is among the Negroes and Italians . . . [in whom] it is not uncommon to see marked rickets in those getting nothing but the breast" (p. 242). By current standards, growth retardation was endemic. The mean height achieved by boys 4 to 9 years of age measured in New York City in 1895 was at approximately the 25th percentile when superimposed on the growth curves constructed from measurements of a national sample of boys measured in the United States in the late 1960s.

THE EUGENICS MOVEMENT IN THE UNITED STATES AND THE SYNDROME OF "HEREDITARY FEEBLE-MINDEDNESS"

At the height of the eugenics movement in the United States, at the turn of the 20th century—two sets of families, the Jukes and the Kallikaks, were used to "document" the hereditary nature of mental retardation, poverty, and antisocial behavior (Dugdale, 1877; Goddard, 1912, 1914; Kevles, 1986). The Jukes and the Kallikaks are always cited together, but they are very different studies leading to very different conclusions.

In 1877, Richard Dugdale published his studies of "crime, pauperism disease and heredity" among the inhabitants of New York state prisons, many of whom were related and to whom he gave the name "Jukes." ". . . . [I]n idiocy and insanity. . . . ," Dugdale notes (1877), "heredity is the preponderating factor in determining career; but it is, even then, capable of marked modification for better or worse by the character of the environment (p. 65). . . . The essential characteristics of [the Jukes] are great vitality, ignorance and poverty. They have never had a training which would bring into activity the aesthetic tastes, the habits of reasoning, or indeed a desire for the ordinary comforts of a well ordered home." (p. 66)

By contrast, Henry Goddard, Director of the Vineland Training School for Feeble-minded Boys and Girls in New Jersey, reported, ". . . . no amount of education or of good environment can change a feeble-minded individual into a normal one" (1913) and "[S]ince feeble-mindedness is in all probability transmitted in accordance with the Mendelian Law of Heredity, the way is open for eugenic procedure which will mean much for the future welfare of the race" (1914, p. 590).

Though the later eugenicists were bigoted in their social outlook and biased in their science, it is likely that they made accurate observations: feebleminded Kallikak parents produced feebleminded Kallikak children. It is well recognized now that Goddard was seeing the cumulative effects of poverty and problems with parent–child interaction. It is our hypothesis in *Malnourished Children in the United States* that nutrition-related disorders, including iron deficiency, lead poisoning, and of most recent concern, in utero exposure to alcohol, contribute (then and now) to the observed transgenerational deprivation and antisocial behavior within these families (see Figure I.1).

Goddard explains this with the same logic which proclaims that a hereditary feeblemindedness causes poverty: "Everything seems to indicate that alcoholism . . . occurs in families where there is some form of neurotic trait, especially feeble-mindedness. The percentage of our alcoholics that are also feeble-minded is very great. Indeed one may say without fear of dispute that more people are alcoholic because they are feeble-minded than vice-versa" (1914, p. 493).

"Perhaps," writes Rosenberg (1974), "the most remarkable aspect of Dugdale's work is the systemic misuse of his conclusions by succeeding generations" (p. 223). The acceptance of Dugdale's positivist attitudes, similar to those of Goldberger, ". . . . could hardly have survived in this climate [of the later eugenicists]: it was in short supply in minds beginning to articulate a growing race consciousness" (p. 224).

Rather than continue the "nature" *versus* "nurture" debates of recent years (Kevles, 1985), it is necessary to investigate how disorders with developmental consequences (such as Fetal Alcohol Syndrome [FAS]) interact with the social environment which produces FAS (alcoholism and poverty) to produce transgenerational poverty—a "nature" *cross* "nurture" model.

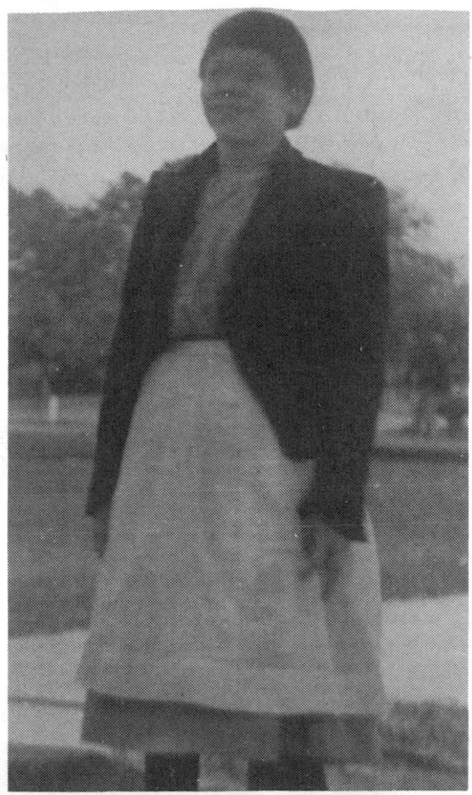

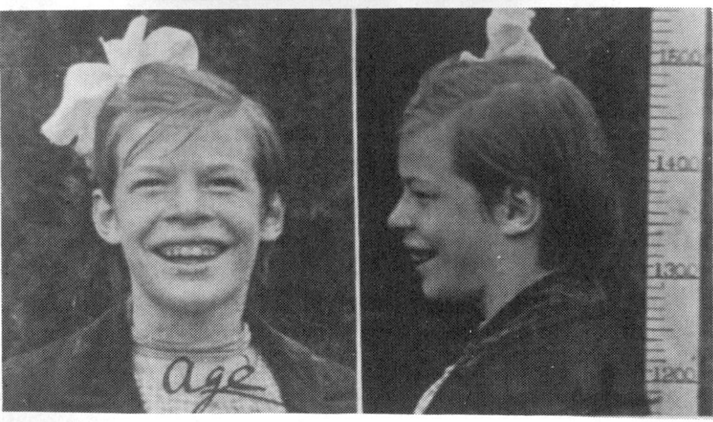

FIGURE I.1 This young woman, Pauline "Kallikak," shows the full effect of in-utero alcohol or Fetal Alcohol Syndrome (FAS). Her parents were "drunkards." She is short; her height is 1501 mm (just less than 5 feet). She is mentally retarded and microcephalic; her head circumference is 515 cm. She shows the major dysmorphic features of FAS including a long upper lip, narrow vermillion border, absent philtrum ("cupid's bow"), and midface hypoplasia with short palpebral fissures (see chapter 10). She is also anemic; her hemoglobin concentration is 9.8 g/dl (see chapter 8).

THE GREAT DEPRESSION REVISITED

During the last election campaign of the 1920s, future President Herbert Hoover made the optimistic promise that all Americans would have "a car in every garage and a chicken in every pot." But the economy of the United States collapsed in October 1929, and, as would be expected, the nutritional well-being of many Americans declined. By July 1930 an alarming increase in the death rate from pellagra was reported (*Journal of the American Medical Association* [JAMA], 1932) with 468 case fatalities among the 1,442 reported in North Carolina in the first 6 months of the year. More than 20,000 persons were affected statewide.

A JAMA editorial from October 1932 responded to the idea that the reduction in overeating of rich food may have beneficial effects:

> While a few adults may be saved by economic necessity from the results of gluttony, the fact that thousands of children are suffering from malnutrition is more important. . . . Too often the social agency has been under fire from unthinking persons, who still regard certain essential foodstuffs, such as orange juice and butter-fat, as luxuries rather than necessities.

In 1933, Alice B. Foote published a plan for "home management [of] house meals at seventeen cents a day." This diet provided about 2,300 calories a day with 75 g of protein, 1.45 g of calcium, and 13 mg of iron per person. Almost half of the calories came from milk and milk products. The daily meat allotment was just under 1 oz of liver with beans and cereal grains being the major source of iron. An extremely low amount of money was spent on fresh fruits and vegetables. As will be shown in chapter 8, children on such a diet would have been at high risk for iron deficiency. This documentation that it was possible to spend minimal amounts of money to purchase the cheapest available foods and suppress hunger laid the foundation for the "USDA-Thrifty Food Plan," which was maintained until the late 1970s when its inadequacy was recognized (Lane & Vermeesch, 1979). Other measures besides a full stomach are required to show nutritional sufficiency.

The growth of children provides the most meaningful indicator of nutritional status (Garn & Clark, 1975). In a depression era report, Palmer (1933) shows growth data for children in Hagerstown, Maryland, a town that "does not represent the most severely stricken type of community." He showed that boys and girls 6 to 10 years of age who received a free lunch or whose families received welfare aid showed a diminution in mean weight from no less than 2.5 lb (girls at age 7) to as great as 7.8 lb (girls at age 11) when compared with other children. This last-noted discrepancy suggests that undernutrition was affecting sexual development among the girls whose families required assistance.

Probably the high point for nutrition studies in the United States, at least with respect to a concern for the needs of the common citizen, came at the end of the Great Depression of the 1930s with the onset of World War II. Aware that the survival of the nation depended on the fitness of its youth, the National Research Council sponsored a series of investigations into the factors influencing the selection of diet and changing food habits to maintain optimal nutrient intake under adverse circumstances. These studies form the basis for the discussion of changing food habits that introduce Part 3.

SILENCE OF THE POSTWAR ERA

Postwar prosperity was not shared by all Americans. Though widespread malnutrition among the poor continued, poverty and malnutrition were not addressed by the general academic community during the late 1940s and 1950s, and funding for such investigations was not available. During that era, scientists in American universities were expected to take loyalty oaths to federal, state, and local governments. The combination of intellectual curiosity and social conscience could be lethal to a professional career. "Excessive" concern for inequities, such as malnutrition of poor children, made one suspect.

CURRENT ERA

In 1962, Michael Harrington published *The Other America*, which documented the extent of poverty in the United States. Social inequity, once again, became a topic of serious study (see Birch & Gussow, 1970) and the target of intervention efforts that have continued to the present day. In 1970, Birch and Gussow reviewed data then available to show that malnutrition was affecting the school performance of children in the United States. Brown, in *Starving Children: The Tyranny of Hunger* (1977), provided data from studies conducted in Mississippi with results comparable to those of children in developing countries.

In the modern era, we have the tools needed to establish the level of malnutrition in the society as a whole. In recent years, three large-scale studies of nutritional status were conducted in the United States. These were (a) the National Health and Nutrition Examination Survey (NHANES), (b) the Ten-State Nutrition Survey, 1968–1970 (TSNS), and (c) the Preschool Nutrition Survey (Owen, Kram, Garry, et al., 1976). They are distinguished for their attention to measures of socioeconomic level, large sample sizes, and vigorous attempts to identify environmental sources of stress that may interfere with growth. The studies are cited throughout this text and provide the most definitive and comprehensive documentation that malnutrition in the United States represents more than isolated occurrences.

Garn and Clark (1975), in their review of the TSNS, conclude that malnutrition in the United States is not of the acute variety seen in developing countries. There are, however, "remarkably consistent socioeconomic effects on size, growth and development that have major bearing on the nation's health and the national welfare." As they write, "The dimensions of poverty are spelled out in the growth of children."

Owen et al. (1974) note that measures of nutritional status considered in the Preschool Nutrition Survey correlate directly with the education and income of the head of household. With respect to anemia secondary to iron deficiency, they found that mean and 5th percentile for hemoglobin level were substantially lower among 1- to 2-year-old children from the lowest socioeconomic status group than among children from wealthier families with better educated parents (see Table I.1).

Today, iron deficiency may be a disappearing phenomena because, in part, of the great success of food supplementation programs such as the Supplemental Program for Women, Infants and Children (WIC) (Dallman, 1986). WIC (and the food stamp program), however, only provide food for half of the eligible families (Stockman, 1987), a phenomenon that increases the vulnerability of poor families to intermittent food shortages, hunger, and malnutrition (Kotz, 1979). Even proven success has not moved the political establishment to assure that every infant is well fed. Those that speak of going back to basics in education should recognize that only a healthy, well-nourished child can learn. The issues surrounding our successes and failures are discussed in the Part 3 of this text.

CYCLE OF POVERTY

It is striking to compare the pessimism of the eugenicist Goddard (1914)—"no environmental changes will help"—with the optimism of the nutritionist Goldberger—"great economic and social advantages [are] to be gained if the cycle could be broken . . ." (Sebrell, 1955).

In modern terminology, that cycle is the "cycle of poverty," the people who are affected are the "underclass," and the behaviors that characterize the people and sustain the cycle reflect a phenomenon referred to, with much controversy attached, as "the culture of poverty"

TABLE I.1 Hemoglobin level and socioeconomic status in the United States, 1968 to 1970

	SOCIOECONOMIC STATUS LEVEL			
	1 (lower	2	3	4 higher)
Mean hemoglobin (gm/dl)	11.6	12.0	12.4	12.5
5th percentile	7.8	9.2	10.2	10.7

(Wilson, 1987; Lewis, 1966). It is, therefore, appropriate to consider the contributions of the cycle of poverty to the occurrence of undernutrition.

Not every child who grows up in a poor household enters the cycle of poverty. No one can say how the presence or absence of societal forces—good or bad—the strengths and weaknesses of family life, and the intrinsic qualities of the child will interact to affect the life of any particular child. But, conditions of prolonged poverty within a community, however, create a "powerful environment"—a persistent set of forces that affect the characteristics of virtually an entire population (Bloom, 1964)—that will result in some of the families becoming part of an underclass. This is the case in the United States today where 5 million children live in poor families (*Five Million Children*, 1990) with an estimated 10% of them (500,000 children) showing inadequate diet, hunger, or malnutrition (Physicians' Task Force on Hunger, 1985).

Malnutrition is a sensitive and specific indicator of the social conditions associated with poverty. It is not an isolated occurrence in the life of an undernourished child. The children and their families that are most affected by poverty are those that have fewer personal and economic resources with which to face stressful situations than do poor families that have better abilities to cope with adversity (Graham, 1985; Karp, Haaz, Starko, & Gorman, 1974; Karp, Snider, Fairorth, et al., 1984; Williams, 1954). The fact that some poor families function better than others, however, is not a credible defense for the neglect of the poor that has characterized contemporary life in the United States (Karp, Fairorth, Kanofsky, et al., 1978; Katz, 1989).

The course of events in this country has been very different from that of the other industrialized democracies. Most developing countries are unable to respond to social dislocation and malnutrition. By contrast, all industrial democracies, other than the United States, have social policies that take advantage of the wealth generated by free-market economies to maintain the general well-being—including good nutrition—of their people. "[C]hildren's welfare is protected because it is viewed as crucial to the children's and the nations' future" (Hechinger, 1990). The close link between economic distress and poor nutritional status demands attention.

REFERENCES

Birch, H. G., & Gussow, J. D. (1970). *Disadvantaged children: Health, nutrition, and school failure.* New York: Harcourt Brace & World.

Bloom, B. S. (1964). *Stability and change in human characteristics.* New York: Wiley.

Brown, R. (1977). *Starving children: The tyranny of hunger.* New York: Springer Publishing Co.

Dallman, P. (1986). Iron deficiency in the weanling: A nutritional problem on the way to resolution. *Acta Pediatrica Scandinavica, 323*(Suppl.), 59–67.

Dugdale, R. L. (1877). *The Jukes: A study in crime, pauperism, disease and heredity.* New York: GP Putnam's Sons.

Five million children: A statistical profile of our poorest young children. (1990). National Center for the Study of Children in Poverty, School of Public Health, Columbia University, New York.

Foote, A. B. (1933). Home management house meals at seventeen cents a day. *Journal of Home Economics*, 479–80.

Garn, S. M., & Clark, D. C. (1975). Nutrition, growth, development and malnutrition: Findings from the 10-State Nutrition Survey of 1968–70. *Pediatrics, 56*, 306–319.

Goddard, H. H. (1912). *The Kallikak family: A study in feeble-mindedness.* New York: The Macmillan Co.

Goddard, H. H. (1913). One man's wild oats. *Scientific Temperance Journal.* January, 51–52.

Goddard, H. H. (1914). *Feeble-mindedness: Its causes and consequences* (pp. 474–492). New York: The Macmillan Co.

Graham, G. G. (1985). Poverty, hunger, malnutrition, prematurity, and infant mortality in the United States. *Pediatrics, 75*, 117–25.

Harrington, M. (1962). *The other America.* New York: Macmillan.

Hechinger, F. (1990, August 1). About education: Why France outstrips the United States in nurturing its children. *New York Times*, p. B8.

Holt, L. E. (1911). *The diseases of infancy and childhood* (6th ed.). New York: Appleton.

JAMA News. (1930, August 16).

Depression death rates [Editorial]. *Journal of the American Medical Association* (1932, October 15), 13.

Karp, R. J., Haaz, W. S., Starko, K., & Gorman, J. (1974). Iron deficiency in families of iron deficient inner-city school children. *American Journal of Diseases of Children, 128*, 18–20.

Karp, R. J., Fairorth, J. W., Kanofsky, P., et al. (1978). Effects of rise in food costs on hemoglobin concentrations of early school-age children, 1972–1975. *Public Health Reports, 93*, 456–459.

Karp, R. J., Snider, E., Fairorth, J. W., et al. (1984). Parental behavior and the availability of foods among undernourished inner-city children. *Journal of Family Practice, 18*, 731.

Katz, M. B. (1989). *The undeserving poor*. New York: Pantheon.

Kotz, N. (1979). *Hunger in America: The federal response*. New York: The Field Foundation.

Lane, S., & Vermeersch, J. (1979). Evaluation of the thrifty food plan. *Journal of Nutrition Education, 11*, 96–98.

Lewis, O. (1966). The culture of poverty. *Scientific American, 215*, 19–25.

Owen, G. M., Kram, K. M., Garry, P. J., et al. (1974). A study of the nutritional status of preschool children in the United States, 1968–1970. *Pediatrics, 53*(Suppl.), 597–646.

Palmer, C. E. (1933). Growth and the economic depression: A study of the weight of elementary school children in 1921–1927 and 1933. *Public Health Reports, 48*, 1277–92.

Physician Task Force on Hunger in America. (1985). *Hunger in America: The growing epidemic*. Middletown, CT: Wesleyan University Press.

Rosenberg, C. (1974). The bitter fruit: Heredity, disease and social thought in 19th century America. *Perspectives in American History, 8*, 189–235.

Schneider, H. A. (1983). Biologic setting of modern nutritional sciences. In H. A. Schneider, C. E. Anderson, & D. B. Coursin (Eds.), *Nutritional support of medical practice* (2nd ed.). New York: Harper & Row.

Sebrell, W. H. (1955). Joseph Goldberger [Biographical essay]. *Journal of Nutrition, 55*, 3–12.

Stockman, J. A. (1987). Iron deficiency anemia: Have we come far enough? *Journal of the American Medical Association, 258*, 1645–1647.

Williams, C. D. (1954, February 13). Self-help and nutrition: Real needs of "underdeveloped" countries. *Lancet*, 323.

Wilson, W. J. (1987). *The truly disadvantaged: The underclass and the inner-city*. Chicago: University of Chicago Press.

Part I
Dimensions of the Problem

Poverty and disadvantage are increasing in the United States. Because nothing will change for the poor if we plan actions based on prejudices—even positive ones—about the nature of poverty, it is essential to define carefully what we mean by poverty, disadvantage, achievement, and success. Part 1 provides a conceptual framework for work with the poor by describing the nature of poverty in our society and the links between poverty and nutritional status, health, and development.

In chapter 1, Johnston and Markowitz ask the question: "Are the data there?" or as they restate it: "Do the data justify action?" Chapter 2 comes from the field of developmental psychology and is written by Wachs. In an earlier work (Wachs & Gruen, 1982), Wachs defined an essential dilemma for nutritional scientists. "It is becoming increasingly clear that nutrition in and of itself may not have major effects upon development unless it interfaces with the child's specific experiential-ecological environment." In this text, he asks how that interface is maintained.

Identifying the consequences of malnutrition is not an easy task. Accusations have been made that developmental tests manifest class and racial prejudice. In chapter 3, Sewell, Price and Karp suggest changing the function of testing away from labeling and placement to assisting in the planning of therapy for infants and young children with developmental problems. They show how multiple environmental influences, including malnutrition, create the circumstances by which malnutrition and poverty in one generation repeat themselves in the next.

The final chapter in this part shows that the dietary practices of poor people are adaptive. The data show that the prevalence of malnutrition is directly related to the national food economy and public policy—or, more accurately, nonpolicy. It is equally demonstrable that the families most vulnerable to ills of all sorts also suffer from malnutrition. Parents in these families lack the skills needed to nourish and nurture children. Under our current national policy, resources are not made available to confront and correct the multiple and interdependent problems faced by the families of the poor.

REFERENCE

Wachs, T. D., & Gruen, G. (1982). *Early experience and human development.* New York: Plenum.

1

Do Poverty and Malnutrition Affect Children's Growth and Development: Are the Data There?

Francis E. Johnston and Diane Markowitz

Poverty is characterized by great need, destitution, and a lack of those things that are essential for life. Though found worldwide, poverty is particularly troublesome in nations in which there is social inequality and a large income disparity between the affluent and the needy. Wilson and Ramphele (1989) note that the existence of poverty is especially significant for four reasons.

1. It inflicts great damage to those who are affected.
2. It is extremely inefficient in economic terms.
3. A high degree of inequality "makes human community impossible."
4. In many societies it is symptomatic of a deeper malaise.

This chapter examines the consequences of poverty as seen in the growth and development of the children of the poor, for whom poverty is seen as constituting a "powerful environment" (Bloom, 1964). A powerful environment is described by Bloom as a persistent set of forces that affect the characteristics of virtually an entire population. The effects are one-way, in that, although 90% to 95% of persons come under its influence, individuals are relatively powerless to alter the environment. In the case of the deprived, there is a downward shift of the distribution curve for any variable that is affected.

The extent to which genetic differences affect growth also may make it more difficult to identify clearly the effects of malnutrition. In the "powerful environment" of poverty, genetically influenced variation in growth potential may be suppressed (Alvarez, Hertzog, & Dietz, 1984; Scholl, Carvioto, deLicardie, & Johnston, 1983). Not until nutrition is optimal in all groups can hereditary variability within and between populations be demonstrated (Bielicki, 1980). In both the developing *and* the developed world, a clear relationship still can be seen between socioeconomic status and growth. With the exception of the Scandinavian states, where most of the population appears to be growing optimally, in most societies there are documented relationships between differences in standard of living and growth.

The detrimental effects of inadequate nutrition on growth and development have been amply demonstrated to be significant, although the degree of the effect is dependent on the degree of malnutrition. Decades of research have proved that the children of the poor are smaller than those of the affluent members of the same society. Is this association strong enough, however, to lead to the conclusion that the nutritionally deficient diets of the poor alone "cause" the deficits of physical growth and mental development that have been observed? Furthermore, do poor growth and behavioral deficits lead to individuals remaining in poverty when they are adults? Is there a feedback relationship between childhood experience and adult performance?

Put simply, this chapter examines the question: Are the data there? Have the canons of proof needed to establish that poverty and malnutrition affect children's growth and development been met? A broad range of studies, employing a variety of research strategies, will be used to attempt to derive an answer to this question.

ESTABLISHMENT OF CAUSALITY IN RESEARCH

The linkage of hunger and poverty with illness and malnutrition should be clear to any concerned health care worker. Illness, poor growth, and decreased scores on measures of cognitive ability have been identified as part of the consequences of malnutrition (Galler, Ramsey, & Solimano, 1984; Martorell, 1985). Nevertheless, clear evidence of prevalence and distribution is required to generate a firm scientific basis for health and nutrition policies designed to break the linkage.

The type of data collected should be specific to the task. If the purpose is to evaluate the nutritional status of a community, cross-sectional data, in which each individual is examined once, will be useful. Cross-sectional data will allow the growth status of a child at a particular point in time to be assessed. The aggregate information provides an evaluation of the children's cumulative "growth history" up to the point of examination.

When the object is to monitor the rates of growth of individuals, however, longitudinal data are more useful, because individual children are measured serially over a period. This permits the calculation of increments of growth between successive examinations. Longitudinal data are sensitive indicators in that they show the rate, or velocity, of growth and not just the size of children over specific age periods. Decreases in the growth rate of young children, often so serious as to constitute growth failure (Scholl et al., 1983), are frequently seen in association with episodes of disease.

Scientific strategy in determining a cause for an outcome (e.g., the rate of growth), however, involves more than illustrating that two variables (growth and the onset of disease) are related in a population. First and foremost, the directionality of change must be demonstrated: This involves demonstrating that *X* varies and that it changes only when the value of *Y* changes (Susser, 1973). During World War II, a famine in the Netherlands was shown to be associated with reduced birth weight, which was brought about by maternal undernutrition. Among pregnant women in their first trimesters during the famine, the outcome was often miscarriage. For those in their third trimesters, the result was more likely to be low birth weight and decreased head circumference; infant mortality was also significantly increased in the first 3 months of life in this latter group. Populations not affected by the Nazi embargo on transport that initiated the famine did not display the same patterns of infant growth and perinatal mortality. They provided a control for the famine-affected group, allowing us to say, with reasonable certainty, that it was the decrease in nutrient intake that caused the miscarriages, the low birth weight, and the higher mortality (Susser, 1989).

The Dutch famine is an example of a good way to model the cause and effect of undernutrition.

Famine → Malnutrition → Poor fetal development

Nevertheless, the usefulness of such a model is limited in explaining the problems we face today in the United States. The Dutch famine was an example of an acute, severe shortage brought on by a specific cause, a shutdown of food shipments into the Netherlands. Conversely, in the United States, we are dealing primarily with chronic, mild-to-moderate malnutrition, in which multiple factors influence each other as well as child development both directly and indirectly. The causal model is less clear and the effects more difficult to demonstrate. In developing nations, where severe deprivation on a wide scale leads to clear-cut outcomes, the epidemiology of malnutrition is simpler to demonstrate. In the United States, most of the growth disturbances seen are not solely attributable to malnutrition. In 9% to 22% of children reported with suboptimal growth, no organic cause can be found. Of these, it is estimated that between 15% and 55% have psychosocial failure to thrive, a condition in which limited social and emotional stimulation and malnutrition have a synergistic effect (Murray & Glassman, 1982).

GROWTH AS AN INDICATOR OF ENVIRONMENTAL ADEQUACY

There are data that indicate the sensitivity of the growth process to the environment. Tanner (1986) has noted that "the growth of children amongst the various groups which make up a contemporary society reflects rather accurately the material and moral condition of that society." In short, the unfolding of adult morphology during the years of infancy and childhood occur within an environment that molds and shapes its expression. Although individual children may differ from each other because of their genotypes, the differences among the means of samples reflects, to a major degree, differences in their environments. Figure 1.1 presents the mean heights of samples of 7-year-olds of high and low socioeconomic class from different genetic backgrounds. It is clear that the differences attributable to variables influenced by socioeconomic status are considerably greater than that associated with genetic background.

The growth status of children, therefore, provides a record of their nutritional and health history. Height and, to a slightly less degree, weight, are particularly powerful indicators because they are measures of overall body size and reflect the accumulation of many small changes throughout the body. For this reason, surveys of children, such as the National Health and Nutritional Examination Survey

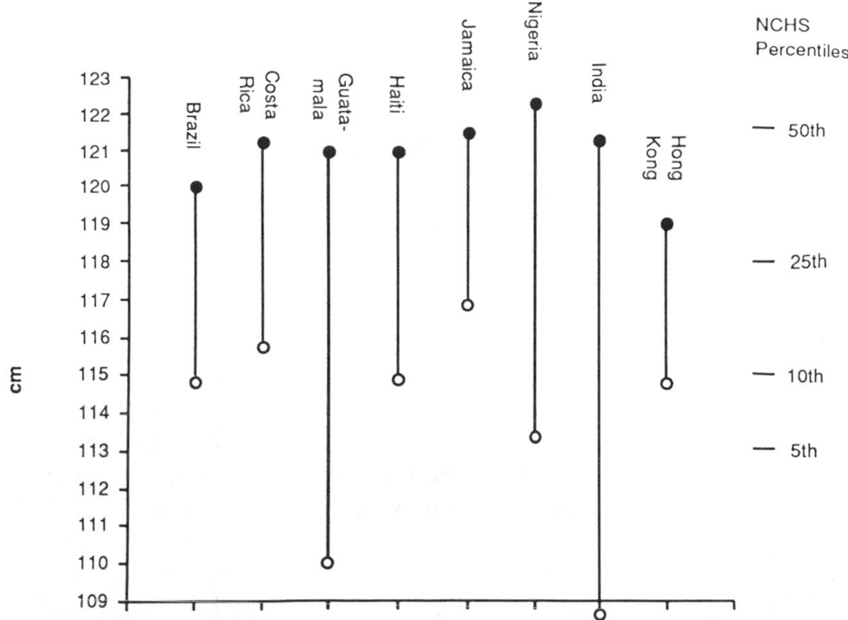

FIGURE 1.1 Mean heights of 7-year-old boys of high (•) and low (o) socioeconomic class.

(NHANES) in the United States, have been used widely throughout the world to monitor the nutritional and health status, not just of the children but also of the entire population. Groups judged to be potentially at risk have been the focus of these studies.

Moreover, just as growth status is an indicator of environmental history, it is also an indicator of functional potential as seen in tests of both cognitive development (Johnston & Low, 1991) and work capacity (Spurr & Reina, 1989). (The issue of learning is taken up in subsequent chapters.) Growth is a mirror of past conditions and a window to the potential for the future.

COMPLEXITY AND INTERACTION OF FACTORS

In the conventional view of science, research is depicted as being conducted in a laboratory setting in which all factors other than those whose effects are being examined are elegantly controlled. Success is largely dictated by the researcher's ability to control possible con-

TABLE 1.1 Effects of environmental factors on growth and development

Cause	Effect
prenatal malnutrition	low birth weight, effect on cognitive ability of infant varies from none to severe
postnatal malnutrition	delayed growth, lethargy, poor socialization,

founding effects, to conduct the experimental procedures with precision, and to measure the results accurately.

Research conducted outside the laboratory, studying children who live their normal lives except when they are measured, is subject to many more problems. More often than not, factors other than the variables studied—which may have confounding effects—cannot be controlled for practical or ethical reasons and must be treated as effects to be measured.

Various factors are known to affect the cognitive development of children. Poverty can be responsible for lower levels of stimulation, malnutrition, and an increased incidence of disease, all of which can directly affect cognitive development. Malnutrition and disease cannot only result in reduced attention span and withdrawal by children but can also affect growth, which, in turn, may reduce the efficiency of learning. Finally, cognitive impairments may "loop back" in the next generation and contribute to a greater likelihood of remaining poor. A systems approach is essential, but it is quite complex, as variables may exert their effects directly, or indirectly through intermediate steps (see chapter 3).

The list shown in Table 1.1 presents the social and environmental conditions that influence growth and cognitive development in lesser developed countries. Similar phenomena occur in the United States with significant consequences to individual children, their families, and society as a whole.

THE UNITED STATES AND OTHER DEVELOPED COUNTRIES

Contemporary problems in the United States are described in the introduction to the text. The 1985 estimate of the Physicians' Task Force indicates that as many as 500,000 U.S. children were malnourished, and the U.S. Centers for Disease Control report that the incidence of low-birth-weight infants rose 2% in the period 1985 to 1987, after a 9% decline during the previous 10 years (Physicians' Task Force, 1985).

Because it is easier to intervene and improve infant and child nutrition than it is to modify parental behavior, the challenge is to discover whether, in the United States, undernutrition plays a discrete role in the genesis of maladaptive behaviors that can be separated from the other components of poverty, a role similar to that found in developing countries. Unfortunately, the complex interactions between poverty, nutrition, and other factors make it difficult to measure the direct effects of malnutrition in developed countries, where malnutrition is usually of the mild-to-moderate variety and is, as noted in the introduction, symptomatic of a deeper malaise in these societies. In affluent societies, however, groups persist that require nutritional intervention, as shown subsequently.

Three Large-Scale Studies in the United States

The NHANES, the Ten-State Nutrition Survey, 1968–70, and the Preschool Nutrition Study (Owen et al., 1976) were described previously. Studies of the rural poor, inner-city blacks, Mexican-Americans living in the Southwest, Native Americans, and migrant workers demonstrate that short stature is clearly associated with poverty in all groups surveyed (Martorell et al., 1987).

Two Community-Based Studies Conducted in the Southern United States

In Arkansas, poor children suffering from nonorganic failure to thrive (NOFTT) were examined and compared with a normally growing control sample of similar economic background. The authors showed that children were able to recover when the families were able to act as a buffer between hardship and the child's immediate environment (Bradley & Casey, 1984). In a similar study in North Carolina, the data suggested that NOFTT among the studied children was caused by both malnutrition and lack of stimulation, and furthermore, that improvement of learning ability is contingent both on nutrition and maternal-child interaction (Ramey et al., 1975).

Intervention that Failed and Why

An unsuccessful attempt at intervention requires mention. In 1969, in Harlem, New York, an interventional trial was targeted toward a population deemed to be at risk: poor, black, underweight, pregnant women (Rush, Stein, Susser, et al., 1980). Because this group was known to have an increased percentage of low-birth-weight babies, and because low-birth-weight babies are more likely to suffer from failure to thrive, it was reasoned that raising the mothers' weight during pregnancy would have a long-term beneficial effect on their infants.

One group of mothers was given a high protein supplement that resulted in an initial superior weight gain among the protein-supplemented group. They then rapidly fell behind the mothers who were given a balanced calorie and protein supplement, as women allowed the protein supplement to take the place of food that previously had been consumed at home. The outcome among supplemented individuals was an increase in premature births, with associated *increased* perinatal mortality. Protein supplements may have placed them at increased risk for premature birth as protein intake exceeded levels now considered safe. Such information was not available to the investigators when the intervention was planned.

This study serves as a reminder that good nutrition policy requires good nutritional science. A thorough understanding of the culture of the people for whom help is intended, in all likelihood, will lead to multidisciplinary rather than solely nutritional interventions. But the basic principle of the study—raise infant birth weight to decrease infant mortality—is correct and continues to drive prenatal intervention programs.

ARE THE DATA THERE?

Without question, the data are there. Poverty is strongly associated with impaired growth and cognitive development, in both developed and lesser developed nations and in all regions of the world where studies have been conducted. The degree of poverty and, just as important, of economic disparity are clearly reflected in the adequacy of growth of the children. We need no more studies examining whether or not the poor are small.

Conversely, there are unanswered questions that need to be studied, and the answers to these questions need to be incorporated into the efforts of planners and public health officials. We need to know why in any poor community, there are those who succeed despite the environmental pressures in the opposite direction. We need to identify specific characteristics and behaviors associated with this "positive deviance," which can be enhanced through interventions designed to improve the standard of living of the people involved. We need to know more about what it means to be locked into the spiral of poverty, from a developmental perspective. Just how disadvantaged as adults are children whose growth, cognitive abilities, and work capacity were impaired by the forces of malnutrition and the stresses of disease? And, finally, how can we intervene in a situation that is socially complex and politically volatile to ensure that children are able to develop in ways that will permit the expression of their genetic potential and avoid the detrimental effects of their environments. Our research needs to be focused more on explaining the mechanisms that act to depress development, and our interventions need to be directed more toward allowing disadvantaged children to grow and develop free of the constraints we impose on them.

REFERENCES

Alvarez S., Hertzog, L. W., & Dietz, T. W. (1984). Nutritional status of poor black and Hispanic children in an urban neighborhood health center. *Nutrition Research, 4*, 583–589.

Bielicki, T. (1980). Physical growth as a measure of the economic well-being of populations: the twentieth century. In F. Falkner & J. M. Tanner (Eds.), *Human growth* (Vol. 3, pp. 283–305). New York: Plenum.

Bloom, B. S. (1964). *Stability and change in human characteristics*. New York: Wiley.

Bradley, R. H., & Casey, P. M. (1984). Home environments of low SES non-organic failure-to-thrive infants. *Merrill-Palmer Quarterly, 30*, 393–401.

Ferro-Luzzi, A., D'Amicis, A., Ferrini, A. M., et al. (1978). Nutrition and growth performance in an Italian rural environment. In L. Gedda & P. Parisi (Eds.), *Auxology: Human growth in health and disorder* (pp. 199–205). New York: Academic Press.

Galler, J. R., Ramsey, F., & Solimano, G. (1984). The influence of early malnutrition on subsequent behavioral development: III. Learning disabilities as a sequel to malnutrition. *Pediatric Research, 18*, 309–313.

Johnston, F. E., & Low, S. M. (in press). *The biosocial ecology of physical growth, cognitive development, and school achievement in a disadvantaged urban Guatemalan community*. Palo Alto: Stanford University Press.

Martorell, R. (1985). Child growth retardation: A discussion of its causes and its relationship to health. In K. Blaxter, & J. C. Waterlow (Eds.), *Nutritional adaptation in man* (pp. 13–30). London: Libbey.

Martorell, R., Mendoza, F. S., Castillo, R. D., et al. (1987). Short and plump physique of Mexican-American children. *American Journal of Physical Anthropology, 73*, 475–487.

Murray, C. A., & Glassman, M. S. (1982). Nutrient requirements during growth and recovery from failure to thrive. In P. J. Accardo (Ed.), *Failure to thrive in infancy and early childhood: A multidisciplinary team approach* (pp. 19–76). Baltimore: University Park Press.

Owen, G. M., Kram, K. M., Garry, P. J., et al. (1974). A study of nutritional status of preschool children in the United States, 1968–1870. *Pediatrics, 53* (Suppl.), 597–646.

Physician's Task Force on Hunger in America. (1985). *Hunger in America: The growing epidemic.* Middletown, CT: Wesleyan University Press.

Ramey, C. T., et al. (1975). Nutrition, response-contingent stimulation, and the maternal deprivation syndrome: Results of an early intervention program. *Merrill-Palmer Quarterly, 21*, 45–53.

Rush, D. E., Stein, Z., Susser, M., et al. (1980). Diet in pregnancy: A randomized controlled trial of nutritional supplements. *Birth Defects Original Article Series* (Vol. 16). New York: Liss.

Scholl, T. O., Cravioto, J., deLicardie, E., &, Johnston, F. E. (1983). The utility of cross-sectional measurements of weight and length for age in screening for growth failure (chronic malnutrition) and clinically severe protein-energy malnutrition. *Acta Paediatrica Scandinavica, 72*, 867–872.

Spurr, G. B., & Reina, J. C. (1989). Maximum oxygen consumption in marginally malnourished Colombian boys and girls 6-16 years of age. *American Journal of Human Biology, 1*, 11–20.

Susser, M. (1973). *Causal thinking in the health sciences: Concepts and strategies of epidemiology.* New York: Oxford University Press.

Susser, M. (1989). The challenge of causality: Human nutrition, brain development and mental performance. *Bulletin of the New York Academy of Medicine, 65*, 1032–1049.

Tanner, J. M. (1986). Growth as a mirror of the condition of society: secular trends and class distinctions. In A. Demirjian (Ed.), *Human growth: A multidisciplinary review* (pp. 3–34). London: Taylor and Francis.

Wilson, F., & Ramphele, M. (1989). *Uprooting poverty: The South African challenge.* Cape Town, South Africa: David Philip.

2

Environment and the Development of Disadvantaged Children

Theodore D. Wachs, PhD

This chapter focuses on the child's psychosocial environment, how it relates to the child's development of competence, and the implications of understanding environmental influences in dealing with children who are at risk for malnutrition. A growing body of evidence indicates that failure to develop competence may predispose to psychopathology rather than psychopathology leading to incompetence (Hobbs, 1982; Loeber & Dishian, 1983). There is also evidence that deviation may be better tolerated by society if the deviant individual has specific competencies that are valued by society (Gold, 1975).

In the past decade there has been an increasing interest in the role of malnutrition in behavioral development (Grantham-McGregor, 1984; Pollitt, 1980). Much of the available evidence deals with moderate to severe levels of malnutrition, which are associated with a variety of deficits in cognitive and social competence. There are fewer data available on the impact of chronic mild malnutrition on preschool and school-age children's development, but the evidence that is available suggests that chronic mild malnutrition is associated with deficits in specific aspects of development, particularly involving attention, alertness, and task involvement (Pollitt, 1980; Rush, 1984). There is also preliminary evidence that suggests that chronic mild malnutrition may also influence school performance (Sigman, Neumann, Jansen, & Bwibo, 1989).

These results suggest the importance of nutritional interventions with young children, but, as Drs. Johnston and Markowitz noted in the preceding chapter, chronic mild malnutrition does not occur in isolation. Rather, chronic mild malnutrition *covaries* with other factors that can also influence behavioral development, such as the characteristics of the child's psychosocial rearing environment (Pollitt, 1988). In practice, this means that where children are at nutritional risk, one must be very careful before attributing behavioral deficits primarily to nutritional risk, because these deficits could just as easily be associated with covarying environmental factors.

This nutrition-environment covariance can be seen in the "striking contradiction" between the developmental outcomes of malnourished children living in impoverished environments and those children living in adequate psychosocial environments who are malnourished owing to organic illness. Pollitt (1988) has observed that children exposed to both malnutrition and psychosocially inadequate environments have a consistently higher probability of exhibiting developmental delay than children living in the same communities without either of these hardships, whereas children whose malnutrition is due to organic illness typically are not developmentally delayed. Given the covariance between inadequate psychosocial environments and inadequate nutritional intake, one obvious implication is that when planning intervention with children at risk for malnutrition, one must consider both nutritional and environmental factors.

But, to understand how the environment can either magnify or attenuate the effects of nutritional risk, we must understand how the environment influences development. The next section outlines some basic principles of environmental action.

NATURE OF ENVIRONMENTAL INFLUENCES

Environment and Experience

First, it is crucial to distinguish between *environment* and *experience*. Environment refers to the *objective situation,* that is, the stimuli, responses, or opportunities a person encounters. In contrast, *experience* refers to those aspects of the environment that *actually influence the development of the child.* This distinction is important because an increasing body of evidence indicates that the same environment will not have the same influence on all individuals. Rather, variation in children's reaction to the environment appears to be mediated by specific, individual characteristics of the child. This phenomena has been called organismic specificity or organism-environment interaction (Rutter, 1983; Wachs & Plomin, 1991). The idea of organismic specificity is not restricted to the behavioral field. Individual differences can be found in responses to drugs, stress, or diet (Rutter & Pickles, 1991).

Documented individual characteristics that mediate the child's reactivity to the environment include *sex of child*, degree of *biological vulnerability* as expressed either through parental psychopathology, or preterm birth, *temperament*, *activity level*, *intelligence level*, and *personal qualities* such as self-regulation, energy level, and stimulus control capacities (for reviews of these topics see Murphy & Moriarity, 1974; Rutter, 1985; Rutter & Pickles, 1991; Wachs & Gruen, 1982; Wachs & Plomin, 1991).

A child's internal working model is one potential individual characteristic which may be of special salience for disadvantaged children. In new situations, children filter incoming information through an organized network of feelings, needs, and expectations, based on their previous developmental history (i.e., the internal working model—Sroufe & Fleeson, 1986). Using children of poor teenage mothers as an example, data from the Baltimore study (Brooks-Gunn & Furstenberg, 1987) indicates that these children have developmental histories characterized by a lack of availability of the mother. Because of both stress and close spacing of siblings, teenage mothers are likely to have low educational aspirations both for themselves and their children. In these situations, it is critical to ascertain what internal working models the children have developed to define both themselves and their world, and how these models influence the child's perception of subsequent experiences such as school or peer relations. This problem is discussed in greater detail by Dr. Bradley in chapter 20.

Transitional Nature of Environmental Influences

During the past 15 years, environmentally oriented researchers have been debating the question of whether or not experiences that occur earlier in life may have a greater impact than those that occur later in life. A satisfactory resolution of this question is found in a recent article by Bradley, Caldwell, and Rock (1988), who report that some aspects of development are uniquely sensitive to early experiences regardless of intervening events, other aspects of development are sensitive to early experiences only because there is a continuity of experience over time, and, for certain dimensions of development, later experiences may be more important than earlier experiences. This suggests that it is more appropriate to conceive of the relation of environment to development as *a process*, involving both earlier and later experiences, rather than as a series of separate critical developmental periods.

Transactional Nature of Environment

The relation between environment and development is basically bidirectional—that is, the environment may initially influence the child, but the child will, in turn, influence his or her environment (Sameroff & Chandler, 1975). Several child characteristics including the child's *intelligence, health status, temperament, nutritional status,* or the *match* between these characteristics and caregiver behaviors, perceptions, or values may have the power to influence the nature of the child's subsequent environment. For example, the child's temperament can influence the availability of food for the child, perhaps through altering the nature of parent transactions with the child (Carey, 1985). Similarly, the child's nutritional status has been shown to predict the quality of the child's psychosocial rearing environment (Sigman & Wachs, 1991).

The Structure of Environment

Bronfenbrenner (1989) has distinguished between multiple levels of the environment, with each level being nested within a higher level like a set of Russian dolls. The innermost level is the immediate environment (or microenvironment) of the child (i.e., the home). Encompassing this inner level is a second level, consisting of the *interrelationship* among the immediate settings in which the developing person participates (i.e., school and home). Encompassing this second level is a third level, which includes settings in which the child may not directly participate but that can affect what happens in the child's immediate environment (i.e., the parents' work setting). The outermost layer is the culture (i.e., a system of shared values, beliefs, and institutions). Bronfenbrenner points out that the child's immediate environment can be influenced by the environment at other levels. For example, external factors distal to the child, such as work stress or neighborhood support may affect the capacity of the caretaker to function effectively with the child. The discussion in this chapter concentrates primarily on the innermost level (the microenvironments encountered by the child), but a full understanding of environmental influences on development must include characteristics of the environment outside the home as well.

Specificity of Environmental Action

Environment-development relations have generally been treated globally; that is, it has been assumed that environment can be characterized as either good or bad, and that good environments facilitate and bad environments impede all aspects of development. However, available evidence indicates that specific aspects of development will be influenced *only by specific aspects of the environment*; that is, a specific aspect of the environment may facilitate the development of a certain skill, be irrelevant in the development of another set of skills, and hinder the development of a third set of skills. This phenomenon is called *environmental specificity* (Wachs & Gruen, 1982).

As one example of specificity, parent-child separation caused by divorce tends to be correlated with acting-out behavior in children, but separation caused by the death of the parent tends to give rise to anxious, withdrawn behavior (Rutter, 1981). Examples of specificity are also found in the nutritional literature. For example, prior research from the Bogata intervention study (Waber, Vuori-Christiansen, Ortiz, et al., 1983) indicates that nutritional supplementation primarily affects motor development, whereas educational intervention primarily influences performance on measures of learning.

Environment as a Covariate

As noted earlier, available evidence indicates that the environment does not act in isolation, but rather covaries with other influences that can also affect development including nutritional status (Grantham-McGregor, 1984), biologic risk (Kopp, 1983), and genetic factors (Plomin, Loehlin, & DeFries, 1985).

There are two implications of this covariance. First, when a child is at psychosocial risk because of economic disadvantage, one must be extremely cautious in attributing behavioral deficits primarily to environmental factors; the deficits can also be due to nutritional as well as biomedical or genetic factors that covary with an inadequate environment. Second, the stronger the degree of covariance among environmental, genetic, nutritional, and biomedical risk factors, the greater the psychological risk for the child. For example, Sameroff and McDonough (1984) report a significant linear relationship between the number of biosocial risks the child is exposed to and the child's level of either cognitive or interpersonal competence; specifically, as the number of biosocial risks impinging on the child increases, the child's scores on both cognitive and interpersonal competence measures decrease. In practice this means that the impact of a single biological or social factor on the child's development may be fairly limited (Rutter, 1981).

Psychosocial Environmental Features That Are Likely to Influence Development[1]

The relationship between variations in the home environment and variations in development is mediated by several factors including individual characteristics of the child, the specific outcome variables and environmental parameters under study, and the role of environmental factors outside the home environment. However, it is possible to detail which dimensions of the psychosocial environment of the child are most likely to influence the development of cognitive and interpersonal competence. Suggested readings include Belsky (1990), Bronfenbrenner (in press), Gottfried (1984), Wachs and Gruen (1982), and Wohlwill and Heft (1987).

ENVIRONMENT AND INTERVENTION WITH HIGH-RISK CHILDREN

Nature of Psychosocial Intervention

Children who are at risk for malnutrition are more likely to have positive developmental outcomes if they are provided with *both* nutritional treatment and environmental intervention rather then just with supplemental nutrition (Pollitt, 1988). For example, an intervention program with fetally malnourished infants (Zeskind & Ramey, 1981) demonstrated that infants who received postnatal environmental stimulation were indistinguishable in cognitive or interpersonal functioning from adequately nourished controls, whereas infants receiving standard medical care alone displayed deficits in cognitive and interpersonal performance through at least 3 years of age. Similarly, research by Grantham-McGregor (1984) on severely malnourished children who received psychosocial stimulation, both in the hospital and after they returned home, indicates that the developmental course of these children was essentially similar to that of adequately nourished children. By contrast, malnourished children who did not receive this additional psychosocial stimulation showed continuing developmental deficits. Although these data indicate that maximal development can be promoted when intervention for at-risk children includes environmental as well as nutritional components, the use of environment as an intervention tool should not be done haphazardly. Rather, to be maximally effective, intervention must be based on *known principles of environmental action* rather than on theoretical speculation about what should work. For example, because environmental influences may cumulate across time (Saco-Pollitt, Pollitt, & Greenfield, 1985), a single time-limited environmental intervention is less likely to produce long-term gains than a continuing series of interventions, each building on previous gains. This suggests the need for a multidimensional process-oriented approach to understanding the interrelationship of environment and malnutrition across time, *before implementing intervention.* In developing a process-oriented approach the following facts must be considered:

1. Malnourished children are also likely to encounter inadequate psychosocial environments.
2. Malnutrition influences children's developmental characteristics, which in turn influence the kinds of reactions the child obtains from significant others in their environment. As Chavez and Martinez (1984, p. 319) write: "malnutrition depresses activity which in turn isolates the mother and family . . . . from all other sources of stimuli that are of vital importance to the functional development of the brain."
3. The child's activity level will influence the way the child processes environmental stimulation (organismic specificity). More active children show better development when left to their own devices, whereas parent mediation of the environment is critical for the development of a child with a low level of activity (Gandour, 1989; Wachs, 1987).
4. It is important to assess which specific environmental factors put malnourished children at risk. For example, for less adequately nourished children the impact of caregiver interaction is primarily on the child's *emotionality and state control* (their own internal sense of well-being). For more adequately nourished children caregiver influences were reflected primarily in the child's *interaction with the environment* (Wachs, 1991). Less adequately nourished children, who receive appropriate levels of caregiver interaction, may develop satisfactorily in terms of dealing with their own internal processes involving state control. However, these same children may develop in an unsatisfactory fashion in exploration or interaction with persons or objects in their environment.

This review of current data suggests the following process model. Children who are low in activity owing to malnutrition may be *more in need of increased stimulation from their caregivers than children who are more active* (Wachs, 1991). However, if these children are reared by caregivers who are also malnourished or, as Dr. Bradley notes (chapter 20), depressed, then these caregivers may be unable to provide the extra stimulation malnourished children may need. Under these conditions the impact of malnutrition on children's development will be multiplicative.

First, these children will be at risk because malnutrition adversely affects central nervous development. Second, malnourished children will have a greater need for active intervention from their caregivers than adequately nourished children because malnutrition leads to lower activity levels. However, the undernutrition of the caregivers may prevent them from providing the extra stimulation these children need—*over and above normal levels of stimulation*—so these children may be at even greater risk for developmental disabilities (Wachs, 1991).

This model suggests that when we develop intervention programs for children at risk for malnutrition, we need to consider simultaneously several variables: the child's nutritional status, the caregivers' nutritional status, the child's behavioral characteristics, the quality of caregiver-child interaction—particularly in terms of the caregivers' ability to provide extra stimulation to the malnourished child—as well as the use of multiple outcome measures across time.

Our ultimate goal as professionals must be to use our knowledge to foster comprehensive programs for developing maximal competence in children, across a wide range of dimensions. If intervention strategies are carried out in a multidisciplinary framework, it is more likely that the gains obtained for children at risk will not only be broader but also more lasting than if interventions are done in small pieces. These issues are addressed in part 3 of this text.

NOTE

1. One notable *omission* from a listing of salient environmental variables is parental socioeconomic or educational status. Recent methodological reviews (Wachs, 1988) have pointed out the problems involved in using these demographic measures as measures of the child's environment. These measures can tell us little about the experiences of an individual child because of the range of psychosocial environments encountered by children *within* a given socioeconomic or educational level. Further, social class or educational level per se accounts for significantly less variability in predicting subsequent functioning than

do more detailed measures of the child's environment. These demographic indices are poor substitutes for more precise environmental measures.

REFERENCES

Belsky, J. (1990). Parental and nonparental child care and children's socioemotional development. *Journal of Marriage and the Family, 52*, 855–903.

Bradley, R., Caldwell, B., & Rock, S. (1988). Home environment and school performance: A ten year follow up and examination of three models of environmental action. *Child Development, 59*, 852–867.

Bronfenbrenner, U. (in press). Ecological systems theory. In R. Vasta (Ed.), *Annals of child development.* Greenwich, CT: JAI Press.

Bronfenbrenner, U. (in press). The ecology of cognitive development. In R. Wozniak & K. Fischer (Eds.), *Specific environments: Thinking in context.* Hillsdale, NJ: Erlbaum.

Brooks-Gunn, J., & Furstenberg, F. (1987). Continuity and change in the context of poverty: Adolescent mothers and their children. In J. Gallagher & C. Ramey (Eds.), *The malleability of children.* Baltimore: Brookes.

Carey, W. (1985). Temperament and increased weight gain in infants. *Journal of Developmental and Behavioral Pediatrics, 6*, 128–131.

Chavez, A., & Martinez, C. (1984). Behavioral measurements of activity in children and their relation to food intake in a poor community. In E. Pollitt & T. Amante (Eds.), *Energy intake and activity.* New York: Liss.

Gandour, M. (1989). Activity level as a dimension of temperament in toddlers: Its relevance for the organismic specificity hypothesis. *Child Development, 60*, 1092–1098.

Gold, M. (1975). Vocational training. In J. Wortis (Ed.), *Mental retardation and developmental disabilities* (Vol. 7). New York: Bruner-Mazel.

Gottfried, A. (1984). Home environment and early mental development: Integration, meta-analysis and conclusions. In A. Gottfried (Ed.), *Home environment and early mental development.* New York: Academic Press.

Grantham-McGregor, S. (1984). Chronic undernutrition and cognitive abilities. *Human Nutrition: Clinical Nutrition, 38*, 83–94.

Hobbs, N. (1982). *The troubled and troubling child.* San Francisco: Jossey-Bass.

Kopp, C. (1983). Risk factors in development. In M. Haith & J. Campos (Eds.), *Handbook of child psychology: Vol. 2. Infancy and developmental psychobiology.* New York: Wiley.

Loeber, R., & Dishion, T. (1983). Early predictors of male delinquency. *Psychological Bulletin, 94*, 68–99.

Murphy, L., & Moriarty, A. (1974). *Vulnerability, coping and growth.* New Haven: Yale University Press.

Plomin, R., Loehlin, J., & DeFries, J. (1985). Genetic and environmental components of "environmental" influences. *Developmental Psychology, 21*, 391–402.

Pollitt, E. (1980). *Poverty and malnutrition in Latin America.* New York: Praeger.

Pollitt, E. (1988). A critical view of three decades of research on the effects of chronic energy mild malnutrition on behavioral development. In B. Schurch & N. Scrimshaw (Eds.), *Chronic energy deficiency: Consequences and related issues.* Lausanne, Switzerland: IDECG-Nestle Foundation.

Rush, D. (1984). The behavioral consequences of protein energy deprivation and supplementation in early life. In J. Galler (Ed.), *Human nutrition, Vol. 5. Nutrition and behavior.* New York: Plenum.

Rutter, M. (1981). Stress coping and development: Some issues and some questions. *Journal of Child Psychology and Psychiatry, 22,* 323–356.

Rutter, M. (1983). Statistical and personal interactions. In D. Magnusson & V. Allen (Eds.), *Human development: An interactional perspective.* New York: Academic.

Rutter, M. (1985). Stress, coping and development. In N. Garmezy & M. Rutter (Eds.), *Stress coping and development in children.* New York: McGraw-Hill.

Rutter, M., & Pickles, A. (1991). Person environment interactions: Concepts, mechanism and implications for data analysis. In T. D. Wachs & R. Plomin (Eds.), *Conceptualization and measurement of organism environment interaction* (pp. 105–141). Washington, DC: American Psychological Association.

Saco-Pollitt, C., Pollitt, E. & Greenfield, D. (1985). The cumulative deficit hypothesis in the light of cross-cultural evidence. *International Journal of Behavioral Development, 8,* 75–97.

Sameroff, A., & Chandler, N. (1975). Reproductive risk and the continuum of care taking causality. In F. Horowitz (Ed.), *Review of child development research.* Chicago: University of Chicago Press.

Sameroff, A., & McDonough, S. (1984). The role of motor activity in human cognitive and social development. In E. Pollitt & P. Amante (Eds.) *Energy intake and activity.* New York: Liss.

Sigman, M., Neumann, C., Jansen, A., & Bwibo, N. (1989). Cognitive ability of Kenyan children in relation to nutrition, family characteristics and education. *Child Development, 60,* 1463–1474.

Sigman, M., & Wachs, T. D. (1991). Structure, stability and covariates of caregiver behavior in two cultures. In M. Bornstein (Ed.), *Cultural approaches to parenting* (pp. 123–138). Hillsdale, NJ: Erlbaum.

Sroufe, A., & Fleeson, J. (1986). Attachment and the construction of relationships. In W. Hartup & Z. Ruben (Eds.), *Relationships and development.* Hillsdale, NJ: Erlbaum.

Waber, D., Vuori-Christiansen, L., Ortiz, N., et al. (1983). Nutritional supplementation, maternal education and cognitive development of infants at risk of malnutrition. *American Journal of Clinical Nutrition, 54,* 496–497.

Wachs, T. D. (1987). Specificity of environment action as manifest in environmental correlates of toddlers mastery motivation. *Developmental Psychology, 23*, 782–790.

Wachs, T. D. (1988). Environmental assessment of developmentally disabled infants and preschoolers. In T. D. Wachs & R. Sheehan (Eds.), *Assessment of young developmentally disabled children.* New York: Plenum.

Wachs, T. D. (1991). Temperament, activity and behavioral development of children. In B. Schurch & N. Scrimshaw (Eds.), *Activity, energy expenditure and energy requirements of infants and children* (pp. 297–320). Lausanne, Switzerland: IDECG-Nestle Foundation.

Wachs, T. D., & Gruen, G. (1982). *Early experience and human development.* New York: Plenum.

Wachs, T. D. & Plomin, R. (1991). The conceptualization and measurement of organism environment interaction. In T. D. Wachs & R. Plomin (Eds.), *Conceptualization and measurement of organism environment interaction.* Washington, DC: American Psychological Association.

Wohlwill, J., & Heft, H. (1987). The physical environment and the development of the child. In I. Altman & D. Stokols (Eds.), *Handbook of environmental psychology.* New York: Wiley.

Zeskind, P., & Ramey, C. (1981). Preventing intellectual and interactional sequelae of fetal malnutrition. *Child Development, 52*, 213–218.

3

The Ecology of Poverty, Undernutrition, and Learning Failure

Trevor E. Sewell, PhD, Vivian D. Price, PhD, and Robert J. Karp, MD

In the United States, children from the poorest and least educated families consistently perform poorly on measures of cognitive ability. The evidence that there are causal links between environmental experience and cognitive ability provides a conceptual framework for educational intervention to enhance cognitive abilities (Scarr & Weinberg, 1976). With respect to *inherent* ability of children, however, we concur with Wachs and Gruen (1982): Measures of socioeconomic status, properly defined, are too broad to label the capability of individual members of any group.

EDUCATIONAL IMPLICATIONS OF TESTING INTELLIGENCE

Use of intelligence tests to determine special class placement has become a central issue in the controversy over testing in schools. The link between special education and intelligence tests can be traced to the very origin of the testing movement. Alfred Binet, who developed the first intelligence test, was commissioned by the ministry of education in France to identify children who were not profiting sufficiently from regular classroom instruction. His emphasis on remedial instruction in special education was the only focus of intelligence testing.

Unfortunately, from its inception in American society, intelligence testing incorporated a political philosophy that emphasized labeling and special educational placement based on the belief in fixed biologic distinctions between groups. The focus of testing and assessment, therefore, shifted from remedial instruction to custodial services. Both race and socioeconomic status have been credited with marking a inheritable deficiency (Gould, 1984; Kevles, 1985) or as described by Frances Galton, "a natural index of ability," by which deviance from the norm could be predicted (Kevles, 1985). The field of eugenics, by which the hereditable characteristics of humans were established as unalterable determinants of behavior and performance, held sway in the United States through the first half of the 20th century. For example, in Philadelphia through the 1950s, children who were slow (now called mild mental retardation) were placed in classes for the "orthogenetically backward" (OB). Children with behavioral problems were referred to as "orthogenetically delinquent" (OD). Other children knew that OB stood for "out of brains." They made the nature of their condition very clear to these unfortunates. The OB and OD labels were by no means restricted to black children. Illiteracy or other signs of poor school performance in sequential generations of poor whites often predetermined entry into the OB classes.

It is beyond the scope or purpose of this text to analyze the various claims to biologic inferiority of a large section of American society. These investigations, among other failings, ignore the studies that consider the life experience of disadvantaged children (Gould, 1984). The nature of early childhood experience is quite sufficient to explain differences in testing whichever type of prejudice is maintained—race/ethnicity or social class. The concomitant occurrence of poverty, lead poisoning, in utero exposure to alcohol, iron and zinc deficiencies and, at times, hunger engender learning failure in all groups of children.

It may be comforting, in a peculiar way, to maintain discredited racial theories, because they allowed societal or personal inaction; however, the general success of interventions that are given time to work provides the best challenge to the validity of these theories.

INTELLIGENCE TESTS AS MEASURES OF COGNITIVE ABILITY

Central to the controversy is the inference that the poor performance by low socioeconomic status and minority children on intelligence tests is a valid index of learning ability (Sewell, 1979). Whether the definition of intelligence is conceptualized as a summation of learning experiences (Wesman, 1968), the capacity to act purposefully and deal effectively with one's environment (Wechsler, 1958), or simply a reflection of a general confusion in formulating an acceptable theoretical position (Jensen, 1980), intelligence, as measured by conventional tests, does not reflect innate capacity. What we call intelligence is a summation of interactions of genetic and experiential factors.

Simply stated, there are no effects of race and social class on the inherent capabilities of children.

UNDERNUTRITION, DEVELOPMENTAL TESTING, AND ACHIEVEMENT

Walker, Walker, and Vorster (1990) have suggested that the consequences of mild to moderate malnutrition in young school children are exaggerated. They point to one study by Richards, Marshall, and Kreuser (1985) of predominantly white upper-middle-class school children where no correlation was found between anthropometric measures (the nutritional variable) and development, aptitude, and school achievement. These are expected results in a well-nourished population of middle-class children (Pollit, Mueller, & Leibel, 1982). These observations do not carry over to disadvantaged populations.

Among the inner-city poor, nutritional status, including anthropometrics, correlates closely with borderline or deficient cognitive and behavioral development (Hepner & Maiden, 1971; Meyers, Sampson, & Weitzman, 1991). The problem, as noted by Hallberg (1990), is that malnutrition among the poor in developed countries occurs in social environments that affect both nutritional status and learning ability synergistically.

In Philadelphia, school-age children with decreased height for age were found to be older than their classmates, reflecting delayed entry into school (Karp, Nuchpakder, Fairorth, & Gorman, 1976). These undernourished children appeared to be of "normal" size and performance by grade (but not by age) when compared with their younger classmates. Moreover, the parents with undernourished children in the school in Philadelphia displayed ineffective parenting behavior likely to diminish both school performance and nutritional status (Karp, et al., 1984).

We looked at five measures of nutritional status (including height and weight), three measures of cognitive function and development (including a standardized test of Visual Motor Integration [VMI]) and a composite measure of school achievement in the children attending this same Philadelphia school. All measures of nutritional status were significantly correlated to school achievement at the $p < .05$ level with a correlation coefficient in a stepwise regression (age factored out) for weight of .45 and for height of .37 (both p values $< .01$). The correlation coefficients with the VMI were .32 for weight and .33 for height (both p values $< .01$) (Karp, Martin, Sewell, Manni, & Heller, 1992).

But, these data do not show that mild to moderate malnutrition "causes" neurodevelopmental delay or poor school performance. In these Philadelphia studies, malnourished children were more likely to live on numbered (long-running, with heavy traffic, no trees, and deteriorated housing) rather than named (short-running, with little traffic and tree-lined) streets. (That is, a child living on 16th Street is more likely to experience the cluster effects of poverty than a child living on Smedley Street.) This comment reflects differences in the condition of housing stock and quality of life on the streets of north Philadelphia. Thus it is necessary to consider the interaction between undernutrition and the environment which produces it.

No single environmental influence creates the conditions that make continued poverty inevitable. Rather, it is the synergism among these influences that keeps the affected child from escaping from the cycle (Cravioto & deLicardie, 1972; Hallberg, 1989).

Figure 3.1 shows the interaction between poverty and five influences on a child's ability to function effectively in society.

Care was taken to make indirect, rather than direct, connections between poverty and effective parenting as well as poverty and learning failure in the child. Ineffective, abusive, or neglectful parenting coupled with drug and alcohol abuse are found at all levels of society. But poor parents lack education and social support, and that lack interferes with their ability to be effective parents. When poverty coexists with social problems not directly related to poverty (child abuse, drug and alcohol abuse), the consequences to the child's ability to learn are amplified; moreover, there are effects of poverty that are directly related to learning failure: lack of parental education, poor diet, and exposure to lead in the environment. One must also consider the generally poor quality of the schools that serve these children and the effect of that educational experience on learning.

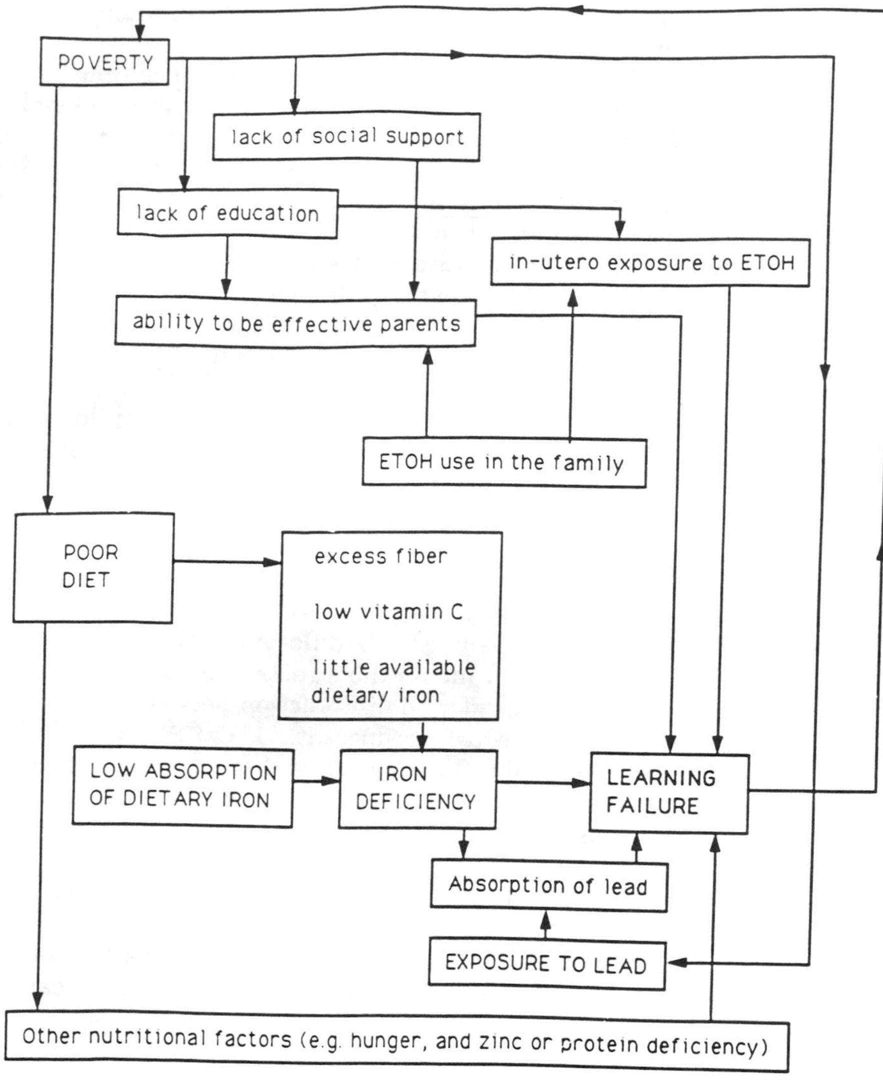

FIGURE 3.1 Ecology of poverty, undernutrition, and learning failure.

Adapted from Cravioto & DeLicardie (1972); Hallberg (1989); Karp, Snyder, Fairorth, et al. (1984). Reprinted with permission of the *American Journal of Clinical Nutrition.*

SUMMARY

The dissatisfaction with tests of disadvantaged children rests, perhaps, not so much with the scientific framework on which intelligence tests were developed, but with the social consequences associated with its uses in educational settings. If the primary purpose of testing is to determine learning potential to facilitate the instructional needs of children (classification and placement decisions), the emphasis on stable, individual characteristics that reflect prior learning experiences is indeed misdirected. It is the link between assessment and intervention that must drive the testing process.

The notion that the assessment of the environment should be factored into the comprehensive assessment of cognitive abilities raises the crucial issues first noted in the introduction: (a) intelligence testing may not be a valid measure of cognitive ability for children whose cultural experiences are marked by deprivations associated with poverty, (b) the preeminent role of the IQ test in the assessment process must be minimized based on relevant information derived from the assessment of the child's environment, and (c) the assessment process must be refocused to emphasize the educational needs of children rather than the labeling and classification goals for which the intelligence test is noted.

It is this conflict between the need to recognize the scientific merits of the IQ test and the clinical demands to contribute to remedial instruction through the assessment procedures that remains the most unsettling issue for practitioners.

REFERENCES

Cravioto, J., & deLicardie, G. (1972). Environmental characteristics of severe clinical malnutrition and language development in survivors from kwashiorkor and marasmus. In *Nutrition, the nervous system and behavior* (PAHO Scientific Publication No. 251). Washington, DC: PAHO.

Gould, S. J. (1984). Human equality is a contingent fact of history. *Natural History, 93*, 26–28.

Hallberg, L. (1989). Search for nutritional confounding factors in the relationship between iron deficiency and brain function. *American Journal of Clinical Nutrition, 50*, 598–606.

Hepner, R., & Maiden, N. C. (1971). Growth rate, nutrient intake and "mothering" as determinants of malnutrition in disadvantaged children. *Nutrition Reviews, 29*, 219–223.

Karp, R. J., Martin, R., Sewell, T., Manni, J., & Heller, A. (1992). Growth and academic achievement in inner-city kindergarten children. *Clinical Pediatrics, 32*: 336–340.

Karp, R. J., Nuchpakdee, M., Fairorth, J., & Gorman, J. M. (1976). The school health service as a means of entry into the inner-city family for the identification of malnourished children. *American Journal of Clinical Nutrition, 29*, 216–218.

Karp, R. J., Snyder, E., Fairorth, J. W., et al. (1984). Parental behavior and the availability of foods among undernourished inner-city school children. *Journal of Family Practice, 18*, 731–735.

Kevles, D. (1985). In the name of eugenics: Genetics and the uses of human heredity. New York: Knopf.

Myers, A. F., Sampson, A. E., & Weitzman, M. (1991). Nutrition and academic performance in school. *Clinical Applications in Nutrition, 1*, 13–25.

Pollitt, E., Mueller, W., & Leibel, R. L. (1982). The relation of growth to cognition in a well-nourished population. *Child Development, 53*, 1157–1163.

Richards, G. E., Marshall, R. N., Kreuser, I. L. (1985). Effect of stature on school performance. *Journal of Pediatrics, 106*, 841–842.

Sattler, J. (1988). *Assessment of children.* San Diego: Sattler.

Scarr, S., & Weinberg, R. (1976). IQ test performance of black children adopted by white families. *American Psychologist, 31*, 726–739.

Sewell, T. (1979). Intelligence and learning tasks as predictors of scholastic achievement in black and white first grade children. *Journal of School Psychology, 17*, 325–332.

Wachs, T. D., & Gruen, G. (1982). *Early experience and human development.* New York: Plenum.

Walker, A. F. P., Walker, B. F., & Vorster, H. H. (1990). Functional significance of mild-to-moderate malnutrition. *American Journal of Clinical Nutrition, 52*, 178–179.

Wechsler, D. (1989). *Manual for the Wechsler Preschool and Primary Scale of Intelligence* (Rev.). New York: Psychological Corporation.

Wesman, A. (1968). Intelligent testing. *American Psychologist.*

Consider a southern farm where the staple food item is pork. Pork consumption by southern-born or originating people, black and white, is twice that of people in the North (see chapter 19).

Any pig raised is likely to be consumed in its entirety. All cuts of pork will be used including the fatty jowls and belly as well as the meaty hocks, loin, and shoulder. The taste for pork will continue when this family moves to the urban North and becomes dependent on the wages of a low-paying job or on welfare payments. But the cuts of meat will differ; it is more likely that the fatty parts will be purchased with less protein and iron, and more fat and salt consumed. Thus, poor urban black families are vulnerable to malnutrition.

By purchasing foods that are usually consumed by the poor, middle-income families "shopping down" drove up the cost of the usual staples for the poor. Poor people were left with fixed incomes and were unable to respond effectively with purchasing power. They had neither purchasing power nor margin for error.

FOOD CULTURE OF CHRONIC POVERTY

One appropriate response of a poor family to the increased cost of food or to decreased purchasing power would be to prepare foods from raw materials, from "scratch." Certainly the use of inexpensive staple items is economical, but in the special circumstances of poor families that are no longer able to prepare food for themselves, one way to save money is to purchase convenience foods of the lowest nutritional value—so-called junk food. To understand a statement that conflicts with everything commonly understood about providing good nutrition at the lowest possible cost, we must look at a food culture of chronic poverty. For in the context of that unique food culture, purchase of foods of the lowest nutritional value is most cost-effective.

Food consumption is not a rational phenomenon. The cost of food, alone, does not cause people to accept foods with which they are unfamiliar. Food selection is based on the culture in which children are born. Food flavor preferences learned in childhood often last a lifetime. The differences between the Eskimos and the Scandinavians, or among the different groups living on various ethnic American diets, reflect differences in food culture. These differences in food cultures can be distinguished by considering four elements (P. Rozin & E. Rozin, 1976; E. Rozin, 1981): (a) the basic substances used, (b) the method of preparation, (c) the food flavorings used, and (d) the social setting for eating. Of these, it is the flavoring systems that label a food culture.

Table 4.1 distinguishes between the characteristics of traditional

TABLE 4.1 Food Culture of Chronic Poverty

	TRADITIONAL From various ethic groups	CHRONIC POVERTY
Basic Substances	meat and/or vegetables pasta and wheat and/or potatoes or rice	starch, fat and sugar
Method of Preparation	raw and/or cooked boiled or baked or fried	"open package" or be served
Food Flavor	spices in combination: garlic, oil, oregano basil, parsley, lemon soy sauce, sesame, pepper burnt onion, paprika dill, garlic	salt, sweet and greasy plus some traditional spices
Social Setting for Eating	(as many as there are peoples in the world) family and friends	isolation

food cultures of different ethnic groups who may be poor and a "food culture of chronic poverty." As will be shown, within a food culture of chronic poverty, there is an economic advantage to the consumption of non-nutritive convenience food.

Almost 50 years ago Kurt Lewin showed that in poor families a kitchen inventory was an accurate way of assessing consumption (1943). In a study in Philadelphia, inner-city families with malnourished children were compared with families where the children were well nourished (Karp, Snyder, Fairorth, et al., 1984). A series of food lists were read to the mothers. These were lists of food requiring

1. Preparation at home by an adult (all nutritious and called "basic" such as meat, rice, potatoes, and vegetables)
2. No preparation by an adult but nutritious (milk, fruit juice, fruit, and fresh vegetables—called "healthy")
3. No preparation by an adult but having low nutrient energy ratios (potato chips, store-bought popcorn, soda, and cookies—called "non-nutritious")

Families were asked: Have you had these foods in the home during the last 2 weeks?

As shown in Figure 4.1, the discrepancies were widest for the non-

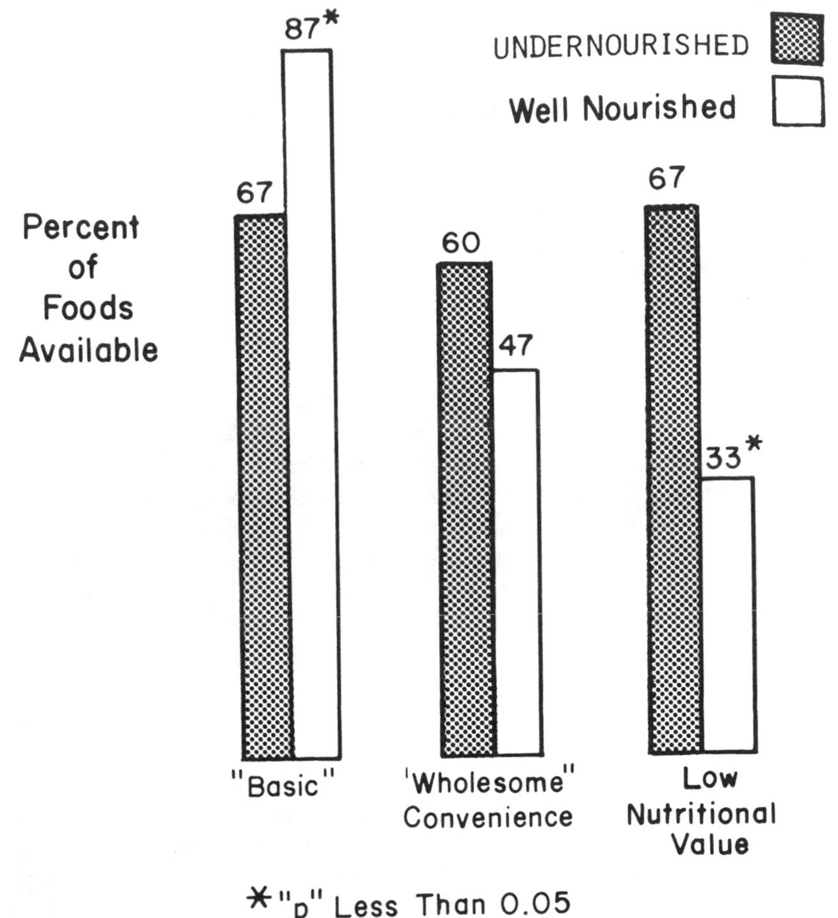

FIGURE 4.1 Kitchen inventories in families of inner-city school children.

nutritious food. In fact there was no overlap. No family with well nourished children had as much non-nutritious food in the home as any family with poorly nourished children.

A similar but not significant difference was found for the availability of nutritious convenience food; there were significantly more convenience foods of all types, nutritious and non-nutritious, in the home of the poorly nourished. Families with well-nourished children used the basic foods to prepare meals.

Most poor people harbor their food resources well, choosing nutritious foods even in the most adverse circumstances (Johnson, Burt, &

Morgan, 1981). The effective response to an increase in the cost of food or to decreased purchasing power is to prepare meals from raw materials; therefore, the use of "junk" food seems, at first, to be an inappropriate and nonadaptive response to poverty. This "food culture of chronic poverty" exists because, for that part of the poor population unable to prepare food at home, sugar and fat-fortified non-nutritious items are the most cost-effective within the choices of convenience foods. The real cost-saving nutritious foods (e.g., rice or beans with some meat prepared at home) are not available.

There is no simple answer to the question: Why do some families become dependent on convenience foods? The poor behave in similar ways as the middle class, and the use of convenience food is ubiquitous in our society. But the same choice for middle-income and lower-income people has a different effect. Poverty produces undernutrition in the common American food culture because of the dependence on convenience foods. Those poor families who are able to respond to their economic condition in a rational way and draw on traditional diets from their own heritage do better than poor families that have acculturated to the convenience food culture of the general society. Thus, most poor families have well-nourished children, but too many do not.

As shown in Figure 4.2, for families dependent on convenience foods (someone outside the home does the preparation), some foods of low nutrient density—such as potato chips and other chip-type snacks—cost less per 100 calories than convenience foods of high nutritional value—fruit juice, bread, or peanut butter—and substantially less than nutritious foods that could be prepared at home by an adult but which are consumed in fast-food restaurants. Foods taken from the United States Department of Agriculture (USDA) low-cost food plan (LCFP) for poverty- and near-poverty-level families will provide adequate iron and other nutrients with the 12 cents for each 100 calories allotted.

Low-cost items from the LCFP—rice, beans, and a little meat—as found in the typical Puerto Rican diet come well below the allotment, but to achieve these savings families require an adult at home who is willing and able to prepare food. Table 4.2 shows a three-day diet from the LCFP.

People will not cross cultural lines just because the nourishing foods of one culture (that based on foods prepared at home) are less expensive than nourishing foods of another (that dependent on convenience). Sometimes this reflects ineffective parenting. In the study of families of undernourished children in Philadelphia (Karp et al., 1984), The Polansky Child Level of Living Scale was used as an indicator of parenting skills and concerns (1978). (The Polansky Scale, as adapted for nutrition-related concerns, is shown in chapter 7 on the growth of

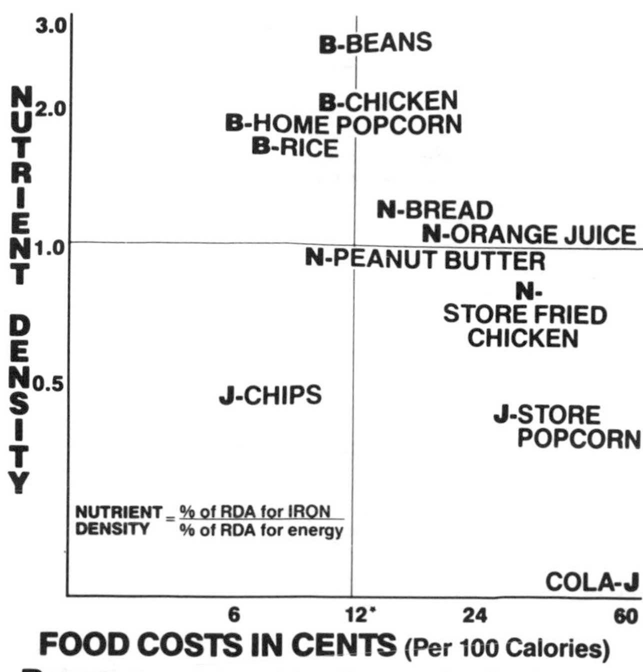

FIGURE 4.2 Nutrient density versus cost per 100 calories for different foods.

disadvantaged children.) With respect to characteristics related to nutritional well being, we observed, Do parents put together balanced meals? Are holidays celebrated with special foods? Is there basic attention to the nutrition of children? For poor families with malnourished children (unlike those poor families whose children were well nourished), the answer was too often, "No." This was one of three studies of undernourished or growth retarded children with similar findings (Casey, Bradley, & Wortham, 1984; Karp et al., 1984; Politt, 1975).

SUMMARY

In this chapter, data from several studies have been used to show two overlapping paths from poverty to malnutrition. The first path is that

TABLE 4.2 "Prudent Diet" for 6-Year-Old Child Derived from the U.S. Daily Allowance Low-Cost Food Plan

3 - 8 oz. cups of 2% (low fat) milk; 2 - 4 oz. servings of meat (1 egg, 1 1/2 oz. beans and 2 1/2 oz. beef); 2 servings of 1/2 cup vegetable, 2 fruits, 5 - 1/2 cup servings grains and cereals. (See Chapter 19 for the construction of nutritious diets for poor families and Chapter 14 for a description of the prudent diet.)

	Calories	Cost in cents Supermarket	local store
Breakfast			
Raisin bran, milk, juice	310	49	67
Lunch			
egg salad with "mayo", bread, lettuce, tomato, milk	429	45	65
PM snack			
banana	105	12	15
Dinner			
rice, meat and bean chili, broccoli, jello, milk	752	91	148
Bedtime snack			
crackers and juice	176	14	19
	1772	$2.11 (12c/100cal)	$3.14 (18.5c/100cal)

of societal neglect of the poor. Food is a commodity to be treated no differently from others. People can eat only what they can afford. By contrast to all other industrial democracies, the concept of planning to support good nutrition among the poor is not a given in the United States. The importance of Women, Infant and Children (WIC) and other supplemental feeding programs cannot be overstated. These are discussed fully in part 3.

It is the question of the quality of parenting, the second path to malnutrition, that is most troubling. For the most part, the food culture of chronic poverty exists in the context of poverty and would be self-limited with the provision of adequately compensated work for parents as well as a public policy of making food available to all children. After all, the use of convenience food is ubiquitous in American society. But the lack of effective parenting in the homes of undernourished children makes correcting the social and psychological consequences of a food culture of chronic poverty a more substantial problem than reversing Engels's law. As Cicely Williams (1954) notes, malnutrition is not due to economic poverty alone but to "poverty in knowledge of the nutritional needs of a child, to defective personal and domestic hygiene, and to fatalism which produces poverty of imagination."

Social issues are difficult to address. The obvious task, learning to prepare foods, has to be considered as part of the process of reintegrating families of undernourished children into society and ending their sense of isolation. These issues are also addressed in part 3.

REFERENCES

Burnett, J. (1976). English diet in the 18th and 19th centuries. *Progress in Food and Nutrition Science, 2*, 11.

Casey, P. H., Bradley, R., & Wortham, B. (1984). Social and nonsocial home environments of infants with non-organic failure to thrive. *Pediatrics, 73*, 348.

Johnson, S. C., Burt, J. A., & Morgan, K. J. (1981). The Food Stamp Program: Participation, food costs, and diet quality for low income households. *Food Technology, 35*, 58.

Karp, R. J., Fairorth, J., Kanofsky, P., et al. (1978). The effect of rising food costs on hemoglobin concentrations of early school age children. *Public Health Reports, 93*, 456.

Karp, R. J., & Greene, G. W. (1983). The effect of rising food costs on the occurrence of malnutrition in the United States: The Engels phenomenon in 1983. *Bulletin of the New York Academy of Medicine, 59*, 721.

Karp, R. J., Snyder, E., Fairorth, J. W., et al. (1984). Parental behavior and the availability of foods among undernourished inner-city school children. *Journal of Family Practice, 18*, 731.

Lewin, K. (1943). Forces behind food habits and methods of change. In *Bulletin of the National Research Council* (Publication No. 108). Washington, DC: Food and Nutrition Board, National Academy of Science.

Polansky, N., Chalmers, M. A., Buttenweiser, E., & Williams, D. (1978). Assessing adequacy of child caring: An urban scale. *Child Welfare, 57*, 439.

Politt, E. (1975). Failure to thrive: Socioeconomic, dietary intake and mother-child interaction data. *Federation Proceedings, 34*, 1593.

Rozin, E. (1983). *The flavor principle cookbook*. New York: Hawthorne Press.

Rozin, P., & Rozin, E. (1976). The selection of foods by rats, humans and other animals. In J. S. Rosenblatt, R. A. Hinde, E. Shaw, C. Beer (Eds.), *Advances in the study of human behavior* (Vol. 6). New York: Academic Press.

Sebrell, W. H. (1955). Biographical essay: Joseph Goldberger. *Journal of Nutrition, 55*, 3–12.

Williams, C. D. (1954, February 13). Self-help and nutrition: Real needs of "underdeveloped" countries. *Lancet*, 323.

Part II
Prevention, Recognition, and Treatment of Nutrition-Related Clinical Disorders

As shown in chapter 4, poverty engenders malnutrition. In part II, the authors will provide ample documentation of the consequences of malnutrition in the lives of poor children. Describing how these consequences create a vulnerability for continued poverty so that poverty and malnutrition in one generation results in poverty and malnutrition in the next generation is the most demanding part of our task.

To make contemporary use of the observations of Goldberger noted in the introduction to this text requires exploration of relationships more complex than many of his successors would care to admit (Sebrell, 1955). We have oversimplified nutritional science. Observations of the responses of starving children to food or of laboratory animals to manipulated diets only partly explain the needs of children caught in what we now call "the cycle of poverty." As the authors in part I have emphasized, no single environmental influence creates the conditions that make continued poverty inevitable. Rather, it is the synergism among these influences that keeps the affected child from escaping the cycle.

As noted in the introduction to the text, the focus here is on the needs of deprived children and, thus, on social considerations. There is, however, within each chapter, a core of information reflecting the underlying effects of nutrients on metabolism and physiology. Good nutritional science leads to good nutrition policy. Most failed attempts to improve the nutritional status of children derive from fallacious assumptions about nutritional needs. For example, the common belief that protein-containing foods are "better" than foods containing fats or carbohydrates is incorrect. As a result, developing countries make plans to raise expensive protein-containing foods that will not feed their entire population (McLaren, 1974). Attempts to nourish pregnant poor women in Harlem may have resulted in protein toxicity to the fetus (Rush et al., 1980). Under the influence of excess protein, calcium needs of adult women climb beyond what is possible to achieve in the diet (Avioli, 1989). From careful study, therefore, a reduction in protein intake has been recommended (Beaton, 1989).

The authors in part II have a common theme. Simply stated, it is easier to prevent malnutrition and its consequences than it is to correct the deficits after they have occurred. In these next chapters, the focus is on the individual child and his or her family. But the clinical concerns of the authors are not considered separately from the environment in which the disorders occur. Clinical conditions are described from several vantage points—basic science, clinical medicine, and social context.

Information is provided for students and professionals expecting to serve children from disadvantaged homes. Thus, the objective is to describe methods for prevention, recognition, and treatment of nutrition-related clinical disorders in the setting of the impoverished family. This introduction concludes with a "nutritionist's checklist" prepared by Laura Dunkely, MS, RD, for her own use at the Pediatric Resource Center at Kings County Hospital.

These problems are not unique to the poor, although the poor are disproportionately affected by many of the clinical conditions described. Three of the chapters require special comment. First, Ajl and Senft have focused their discussion of infant feeding (chapter 5) on the changes in health care delivery needed to reestablish breast-feeding as a community norm among the poor. This is a large topic worthy of a text of its own, and information on routine practices are well presented in the articles and texts cited by the authors. But the changes in attitudes and behaviors that encourage and foster breast-feeding—whether it is the health profession considering the mother and infant or the mother considering her own infant—are the changes needed to reconstruct disconnected families in disadvantaged communities. The benefits of a choice to breast-feed are as important as the benefits of providing breast milk itself.

Chapter 9 by Harris and colleagues extends our concern well beyond treatment of nutrition-related clinical disorders to lead poisoning. Children consume lead because lead is in their environment not because of any genetic precursor, decision of the parent, or choice of diet. With lead-poisoned children, the role of the health care provider, as the authors make clear, is that of an advocate for the poor more than a clinician.

Finally, the chapter on teen pregnancy by Scholl and colleagues has a message that contradicts the currently accepted literature on this subject. Young girls can become pregnant before they complete their own growth. Thus they are vulnerable to undernutrition themselves.

REFERENCES

Avioli, L. V. (1989). Calcium and phosphorus. In M. E. Shills & V. Young (Eds.), *Modern nutrition in health and disease* (6th ed., pp. 142–158). Philadelphia: Lea & Febiger.

Beaton, G. H. (1989). Criteria of an adequate diet. In M. E. Shills & V. Young (Eds.), *Modern nutrition in health and disease* (6th ed., pp. 649–665). Philadelphia: Lea & Febiger.

McLaren, D. S. (1974). The great protein fiasco. *Lancet, 2*, 93–96.

Rush, D. E., Stein, Z., Susser, M., et al. (1980). Diet in pregnancy: A randomized controlled trial of nutritional supplements. In *Birth defects original article series* (Vol. 6). New York: Liss.

Sebrell, W. H. (1955). Biographical essay: Joseph Goldberger. *Journal of Nutrition, 55*, 3–12.

PEDIATRIC RESOURCE CENTER NUTRITION ASSESSMENT

Diagnosis____ WT_____ %ile_____ HT______ %ile______

WT/HT %ile______ IBW______ %______ Failure to gain wt in ____ mos. Recent wt change of_______

Lab Values___________________________ Medication_______________________________

Supplements___________________________________

24 HOUR RECALL: List all foods eaten within the last 24 hours.

MORNING 6:00 a.m. - 11:30 a.m.	**AFTERNOON (12:00 p.m. - 5:00 p.m.)**	**EVENING (6:00 p.m. - 5:30 a.m.)**

FOOD FREQUENCY CHECKLIST: [Indicate frequency per day (d), week (w), or month (m), i.e. 2/d]

I. Milk	Canned fish.....______	Fruit Juice.........______	Butter/Marg.....______
Milk.....______	Canned Meat.....______	**V. Breads**	Sal Dress'g/Mayo______
Cheese...______	Peanut Butter...______	Cereal.............______	Fried Foods.....______
Ice Cream______	Cold Cut/Frank..______	Breads/Rolls........______	Chips/Pretzel...______
Yogurt...______	Dried Peas/Beans______	Pancakes/Waffles.....______	Salt...........______
Puddings.______	**III. Vegetables**	Potato.............______	Catsup/Mustard..______

II. Meats

Beef....._____

Poultry.._____

Fish....._____

Pork....._____

Lamb/Veal_____

Goat....._____

Liver...._____

Green Leafy Veg._____

Dark Yellow Veg._____

Other Veg......_____

Raw Veg........_____

IV. Fruits

Citrus Fruits..._____

Other Fruits...._____

Prunes/Raisins.._____

Rice/Noodles........_____

Crackers............_____

Biscuits/Muffins....._____

VI. Other

Sugar/Jelly/Syrup...._____

Soda................_____

Cookies/Cakes/Pastries_____

Candy..............._____

Gravy.........._____

Pickles........_____

Coffee/Tea/Cocoa_____

Alcohol........_____

Other.........._____

Ethnicity _____________ Food Allergies/Idiosyncracies _____________________

Watches T.V. Y_____ N_____ # of hours_____ Eats when watching T.V. Y_____ N_____ Fear of fat or cholesterol Y_____ N_____ Favorite Snack_____________ Trouble chew'g/swallow'g Y_____ N_____

Feeds self Y_____ N_____ Breast feeds Y_____ N_____ Bottle feeds Y_____ N_____ Uses *Cup*/Glass Y_____ N_____

Comments____

____

____

Assessment____

____

____

____

____

____

Plan____

____

5

Infant Feeding Practices

Steven Ajl, MD, and Carl Senft, MS

In almost every instance, comparing breast- with bottle-feeding gives advantage to the breast-fed infant—less infection, fewer allergic responses, better iron status, closer relationship with the mother, and improved development. Yet, in the first half of this century there was a steady decrease in the percentage of mothers breast-feeding. Then, in the 1960s, there was a surge in the number of mothers in the United States who chose to breast- rather than bottle-feed. But the shift occurred primarily among more educated women and was accompanied by a fall in breast-feeding by disadvantaged women (Faden & Gielsen, 1986).

Speculation surrounds the reasons for the disparity that continues to this day. It has been suggested that low-income women, deficient in language or communication skills, cannot take advantage of information about the health benefits associated with breast-feeding (Miara & Doyle, 1985). In addition, these disadvantaged women who may be aware of the health benefits, lack the knowledge to breast-feed properly having lost their support group—family and friends with experience (Winikoff, Lauharan, Myers, & Stone, 1986). They do not receive adequate advice and guidance from their physician or other health professionals (Lawrence, 1989). Health care providers need to acquire skills to (a) act as a help, rather than a hinderance, to breast-feeding in a population that is unlikely to breast-feed; (b) give support to mothers who bottle-feed their infants; (c) inform all mothers and families that may not have a particularly good diet themselves about the process of transition to solid feedings, (d) address structural impediments to educating new mothers properly.

The clinician should encourage breast-feeding in any woman who is so inclined. Whatever the mother's decision, however, it must be respected. Each case should be viewed individually and proper feeding guidelines set, based on the mother's choice, as it is in the nurturing and nourishing of infants that the process of raising a healthy child begins.

BREAST-FEEDING

Breast Is Best for Human Infants

Successful bottle-feeding is a very recent phenomenon in human experience. Until the 1920s, the technology was not available to manufacture a satisfactory substitute for human milk. A full description of specific characteristics of breast milk, those of manufactured infant formulas, and the vitamin and mineral needs of new-born infants can be found in texts currently available (Barness, 1992; Finberg, 1987)

Bonding Between Mother and Infant. Although breast-feeding alone does not create the special mother–child bond, the choice to breast-feed may introduce and enhance a better relationship between the mother and her infant (Klaus & Kennel, 1976). This phenomenon may prove significant in enabling disadvantaged mothers to feel closer to their new, vulnerable babies.

Improved Developmental Outcome. In themselves, the marked social differences between families who choose to breast-feed and those who do not would predict improved developmental scores for breast-fed infants. In one study of low-birth-weight infants, however, Morley, Cole, Powell, and Lucas (1988) found "a 4.3 point advantage remained after adjusting for demographic and perinatal factors" for babies whose mothers chose to breast-feed as compared with infants of mothers who did not. This seemingly small advantage of 4.3 points is of great importance when considered in the context of the similar decrements in developmental scores associated with other nutritional problems of disadvantaged children (see chapters 3 and 9).

Feeding of Human Milk Limits Infections. Breast-feeding has had a critical role in the prevention of gastroenteritis in the developing world (Unni & Richard, 1988). There are anti-infective elements in human milk that are not present in formula including lactoferrin, the immunoglobulins IgG and secretory IgA, as well as lysozyme.

There is greater protection from infection for breast-fed babies (Chandra, 1979).

Potential for Reduced Allergic Response. Breast-feeding the infant with a strong family history of allergy may reduce the occurrence of atopic rashes, and gastrointestinal and respiratory problems during the first year of life (Fallot, 1980). Chandra (1979) has shown that breast-fed infants have diminished levels of IgE, suggesting that they are challenged less by substances that they see as foreign.

Other advantages include the convenience of breast-feeding and the restoration of the nursing mother to her prepregnant state (Greene, Smiciklas-Wright, Scholl, & Karp, 1988). Extra weight gained during pregnancy is used for milk production. Thus, the return to baseline weight occurs more rapidly when the mother breast-feeds. Breast-feeding serves as a population control device for a community as fertility rates are reduced, but no individual should depend on nursing to prevent pregnancy (Perez, 1972). Changes in consistency and flavor during breast-feeding may serve as an appetite-control mechanism that is absent in homogenous artificial feedings (Worthington-Roberts, & Vermeesch, 1981).

Differences in Growth Patterns. Recently, Dewey, Heinig, Nommsen, et al. (1992) have shown that breast-fed infants weigh less from 3 to 18 months of age when compared with formula-fed infants. There are, however, no differences in length or head circumference measurements. The authors warn that when the growth of breast-fed infants is plotted "they often appear to be 'faltering' after the first 2 or 3 months, even if they are healthy and thriving." Appropriate guidance for breast-fed infants showing this pattern is that the growth is normal, breast milk is adequate, and complementary foods or formulas should not be added.

Who Breast-Feeds?

Breast-feeding in the United States reached a low point in 1971, with only 25% of all new mothers using their own milk to nourish their infants. The highest incidence of breast-feeding occurs among more educated white women, but not for black women where level of education does not seem to affect the rate for breast-feeding (Ford & Labock, 1990; Kurinji, Shiono, & Rhoads, 1988). By contrast, the lowest proportion of U.S. women who breast-feed are those under the age of 20, grade-school educated, lower income, black, and living in the southeastern United States (Report of the Surgeon General, 1984).

For the most part, the black community has not shared in the renewed interest in breast-feeding. The differences between breast-feeding prevalence of black and white mothers seems to reflect cultural differences between the separate communities as well as a lack of support systems such as La Leche League. The factors influencing black and white women of similar economic and intellectual background to breast-feed may differ. Ford and Labock found that for black infants, being sent to a high-risk or intensive care nursery increased their likelihood of being breast-fed while special care had the opposite effect for white infants. Kistin, Benton, Rao, and Sullivan (1990) have recently shown that educational efforts integrated into prenatal care can increase the rate of low-income black mothers choosing to breast-feed.

Bradley notes in chapter 20 that stable black families have within them a "pivotal" person who "serves as the resource of culture, values, beliefs and information, as well as psychological sustenance. Bradley suggests that health care providers make an attempt to identify and then meet the pivotal person. He or she will then become an ally in the mutual transmittal of information from provider to family about health needs, and from family to provider about the cultural traditions of the family.

Barriers to Breast-Feeding Among the Poor

There are considerable barriers to breast-feeding among poor and disadvantaged families. These include lack of education, a nonsupportive family or community, and uninformed health care providers linked to a health care system that does not provide adequate resources for the poor. There is, at present, no process for providing support to the poor or disadvantaged mother who would like to breast-feed.

Lack of Supportive Community of Breast-Feeding Mothers. The best source of information for the intimate topic of breast-feeding is the community of people around the mother. In many communities, the general level of knowledge about breast-feeding practices is quite low. Bottle-feeding and not breast-feeding is self-perpetuating and can be characterized by the 38-year-old grandmother who did not breast-feed and has a 17-year-old daughter with a new baby. Encouragement and support for breast-feeding in such a situation is unlikely; the grandmother is not in a position to offer advice to the new mother having never breast-fed herself. Although most educated white women in their 20's and 30's have mothers who did not breast-feed, the void has been filled by semivolunteer groups like La Leche League.

Lack of Supportive Community of Health Care Providers. Many poor people receive care in busy, overcrowded, stressed prenatal clinics where there is a lack of continuity of care and little concern for method of feeding. After birth, the care may not support breast-feeding (e.g., bottles of formula are placed into bassinets, and mothers do not have 24-hour access to their babies) (Frank, Wirtz, Sorenson & Heeren, 1987).

A health care practitioner should examine the breast-fed infant at 2 weeks of age to check the adequacy of weight gain, and to be sure the infant is wetting his or her diaper often. These are the indications that breast-feeding is going well. For babies not seen until 6 to 8 weeks of age, those mothers who have started to breast-feed often convert to formula use. Careful follow-up must be built into the plans for patient care. La Leche League or similar support networks for breast-feeding mothers should be available.

Support for the Breast-Feeding Mother

The myths and misinformation concerning breast-feeding should be dispelled before delivery. A mother inclined to bottle-feed should never be made to feel guilty or inadequate about her choice, but she should be informed about breast-feeding to ensure that an educated decision is being made.

The position of the child and mother are very important in proper breast-feeding. The baby should first be placed on her back on her mother's lap, with the head on the side from which the mother intends to breast-feed. The baby should be lifted up and brought close to the mother's breast. The child should be turned 90 degrees so that the mother's abdomen or chest and the baby's abdomen or chest are proximate to each other. This will facilitate the baby being able to grasp the areola and compressing the underlying sinuses when she starts to feed.

The newborn should then be allowed to feed on demand for up to 10 minutes on each breast. This may be repeated as often as every 2 or 3 hours. There is no evidence to show that increasing the time per breast from 5 minutes the first day, to 10 minutes on day 2, and 15 minutes on day 3 will decrease nipple soreness.

When the mother and baby go home, usually at about 48 hours of age, encouragement to continue breast-feeding should be offered. To increase the mother's fluid intake, it is recommended that she have something to drink every time she feeds the baby. As noted previously, the breast-fed infant should be seen at 2 weeks of age for a weight check and general assessment.

Common Problems with Breast-Feeding

Somewhere between 48 and 72 hours after birth most women's milk comes in; their breasts will enlarge and become firmer. This process is referred to as engorgement, which is a definite sign to feed baby.

Sore nipples tend to get sorer even as the problem resolves. Assess the baby's position at feeding. If the baby is repositioned so that proper latching on has occurred, sucking will hurt less. Beware of prolonged unnecessary feedings. At times, milk may not be draining very well because of a clogged duct. This will cause mild soreness in one area of the breast that lacks warmth, but shows extreme tenderness, redness, or systemic signs. Sometimes gentle massage over that area and moving the baby slightly will be helpful.

In general, mild illness in the mother is not a contraindication to breast-feeding if she is not taking inadvisable medications (American Academy of Pediatrics, 1983; Lawrence, 1989).

Intervention Strategies Detrimental to Breast-Feeding

At times, gift packs containing formulas are given to new mothers by hospitals before discharge. This practice poses a threat to the duration of breast-feeding. Recently, a major manufacturer of infant formula has initiated an advertising campaign in the local media. This practice is condemned as it undermines the effort to make breast-feeding preferred.

WIC and Breast-Feeding

Recently, Ryan, Rush, Krieger, and Lewandowski (1991) have shown a substantial decline in breast-feeding rates among all segments of society with the decline being "greater among those enrolled in the Women, Infant and Children [WIC] program (compared with those not enrolled)." (See Figure 5.1.) The WIC program (Tognetti, Hischman, & McLaughlin, 1991) challenge their conclusions. The most important issue, however, was not addressed: how to use the economic power of WIC to increase the number of breast-feeding mothers in poor communities.

As will be shown in chapter 18, the relationship between poverty and malnutrition is governed by Engels's law: as food costs rise, foods characteristic of higher income levels disappear from the diet. Supplementary programs reverse Engels's law by providing nourishing foods and by sparing money to be set aside for the purchase of better quality food. With current WIC policies, poor families are asked to choose between a supplement saving them $2.60 in food costs for formulas or

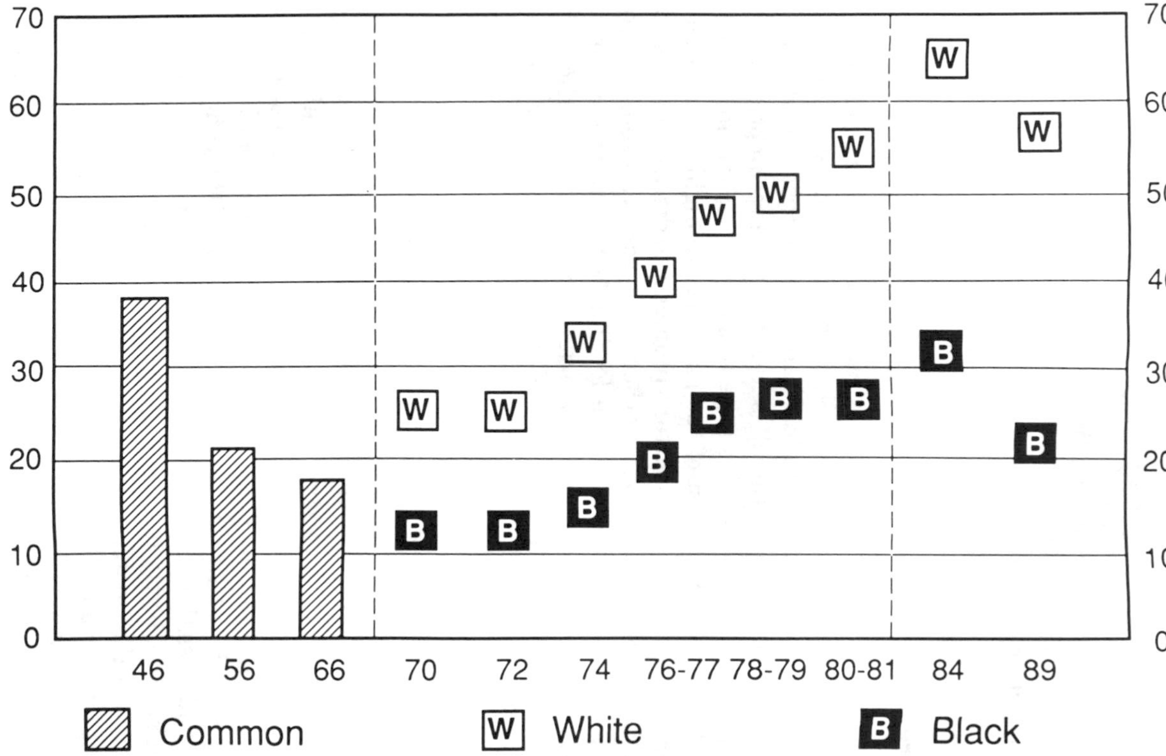

FIGURE 5.1 **Incidence of breast-feeding in the United States. Percentage of infants breast-fed by race, 1970–1989.**

$0.50 worth of food for the mother who breast-feeds. The "bottle option" would seem better even without the known resistance to breast-feeding in disadvantaged communities (Faden & Gielsen, 1986).

The solution is rather straightforward. Rather than being penalized for choosing to breast-feed, WIC mothers choosing that option should be given a food voucher for the full value of the formulas that they have rejected. The role of the parents as both nurturers and nourishers of their children would be enhanced. These issues are discussed in part 3.

The Breast-Feeding Clinic

Breast-feeding clinics have been established at some large urban hospitals. At discharge from the hospital, all mothers who elect to breast-feed are invited to attend the clinic. There is no charge; no one is billed for the visits, and no appointment is needed. The presumption is that many, if not most, of the mothers have little or no support for their decision to breast-feed. But most of the patients are highly motivated to breast-feed, but many have important problems to discuss—babies who could never get onto the breast; mothers with sore, cracked, blistered nipples; as well as mothers who are feeding babies from both breast and bottle. The clinicians are taught to deal sensitively with these and a host of other issues (Faden & Geilsen, 1986; Freed, Landers, & Schanler, 1991).

BOTTLE FEEDING OF BABIES

There are three important changes that have occurred in contemporary life because of the successful formulation of human milk substitutes. First, fathers are able to feed their infants. Second, mothers can leave home to go to work. Third, adoption of infants is possible for the general public. Pediatric text books from the turn of the century until the 1920s address this last problem with comments on the selection of a wet nurse. But bottle feeding requires important technological advances beyond the production in a factory of a chemically acceptable substitute for human milk. A bottle-fed infant will fail to thrive unless the five conditions listed in Table 5.1 are met.

Because the formula-fed infant's intake is regulated by the mother instead of by the baby as in breast-feeding, it is important to teach the mother how to control the baby's intake. Baby feedings are quite variable. In early infancy, a baby will eat 6 to 10 times a day and consume 2 to 3 ounces at each feeding. At 1 month, the number of feedings de-

TABLE 5.1 Bottle Feeding Requires

1. a formula that meets conditions for nutritional adequacy
2. a water supply that is clean and readily available.
3. an ability to refrigerate prepared formulas, and
4. a willingness and ability to clean nipples and bottles.
5. The mother, or the person who assumes that role, must be able to compensate for the inherent nurturing quality that comes with the process of breast-feeding.

creases from 8 to 5, and the intake of one feeding increases from 4 to 5 ounces. By 3 to 4 months of age, most babies are feeding 4 to 5 times in 24 hours and are taking 6 to 7 ounces at each feeding.

The cow-based formulas are sufficiently similar to use as substitutes for each other without regard to brand name. Unfortunately, there are still "low-iron" as well as appropriate iron preparations available. Although newborns do not need the extra iron in the higher-iron–containing formulas until they are about 3 to 4 months of age, start babies on an iron-fortified formula at birth, because it is very difficult to convince mothers to switch types of formula. There is also a strongly prevalent belief that iron-fortified formulas cause constipation, a belief that has been disproved in carefully controlled studies (Nelson, 1988).

Formula comes in several preparations—ready to feed, a concentrate to be diluted with water, and a powder. It is essential to teach appropriate preparation technique. Families may overly dilute formulas to save money. This may result in the failure-to-thrive syndrome.

Evaporated milk formulas (at $0.60 for a 12-ounce can) are used mostly by the poor through the first year of the child's life. (Commercial formulas cost at least $2.60 for each 12-ounce can.) The proper dilution of evaporated milk is 12 ounces of concentrate to 17 ounces of water, and two tablespoons of table sugar. This formulation can be found in older textbooks of pediatrics and is known by many grandmothers. Some mothers will make a 1:1 dilution of evaporated milk that creates a potential for hypernatremia with gastroenteritis among infants under 6 months of age. Unscrupulous merchants have been known to give mothers a kickback to accept evaporated milk instead of manufactured formulas. All children on evaporated milk formulas require vitamin C and iron supplementation as iron deficiency is the usual consequence of using this formula (American Academy of Pediatrics, 1985).

Unacceptable formulations include milk made from condensed cow milk, often used in cooking, and non-dairy creamers that are used as a milk substitute. There are several inadequate substitutes used by food-cult families also.

TRANSITION TO SOLID FEEDINGS—THE USE OF "BEIKOST"

In the Third World, nutritionists emphasize the importance of foods specifically reserved for the infant during the period of weaning (American Academy of Pediatrics, 1980). These weanling foods are referred to as beikost. The concept is as important as the food itself. In developing countries, within large families, the younger children display kwashiorkor—meaning weanling's disease when translated directly— because the protein- and calorie-rich foods needed by the infant are taken by the older children. By reserving a food for weanling children, the older children are discouraged from this practice.

In the United States, beikost is provided commercially and may be begun at 4 months of age. It is unlikely that an older child will take infant cereal or jarred vegetables from a baby. Thus, within reasonable limits, purchasing supplemental foods is recommended. Alternatively, if the family has the resources to prepare clean nutritious food, a home beikost can be made with a clear statement to older children that this is food for babies.

Nevertheless, the disadvantage of home-prepared beikost should be noted. These are (a) parents adding salt and sugar to suit adult taste; (b) overboiling, thus destroying water-soluble vitamins, (c) the chance for bacterial contamination with the large volumes of food prepared, the long "cool-down" period after preparation, and the attempts to keep the food for too long a period. With commercial beikost, powdered infant cereals are iron and vitamin enriched, jarred foods are prepared with minimal salt and sugar, and foods likely to promote allergy are restricted.

The introduction of beikost (foods other than human milk or formulas fed to infants) is not recommended before 4 months of age. Before this age, the introduction of beikost might resemble a form of forced feeding and will increase the chance of choking or, at minimum, overfeeding. It is reasonable to expect that an infant will consume 30% of his or her calories as beikost by 6 months of age with 50% of calories from nonmilk foods by 1 year of age. Foods should be introduced one at a time without mixing, and foods likely to promote allergy (i.e., egg white and wheat) or that can obstruct the trachea (i.e., grapes, nuts, bread, hot dogs, or peanut butter on a spoon) should be restricted. These foods should not be a part of the infant diet.

SUMMARY

The focus of this chapter has been on the provision of support to mothers and families so that the tradition of breast-feeding may be reinstituted across the spectrum of society. The significant improvement in developmental outcome at 18 months of age shown by Morley et al. (1988) among low-birth-weight, breast-fed infants justifies this focus for a chapter written on the feeding of disadvantaged infants. With all of the compelling information on the advantages of breast milk, it may be that the choice to breast-feed is the factor that contributes the most to disadvantaged children. The process itself may be as important as the product.

REFERENCES

American Academy of Pediatrics, Committee on Drugs. (1989). Transfer of drugs and chemicals into human milk. *Pediatrics, 84*, 924–936.

Barness, L. (1992). Nutrition. In Behrman (Ed.), *Nelson: Textbook of Pediatrics* (14th ed.) (p. 105). Philadelphia: Saunders.

Chandra, R. K. (1979). Prospective studies of the effect of breast-feeding on incidence of infection and allergy. *Acta Paediatrica Scandinavica, 68*, 691–694.

American Academy of Pediatrics Committee on Nutrition. (1980). On the feeding of supplemental foods to infants. *Pediatrics, 65*, 1178–1181.

American Academy of Pediatrics Committee on Nutrition. (1985). *Pediatric nutrition handbook* (2nd ed., pp. 37–48). Elk Grove Village, IL: American Academy of Pediatrics.

Dewey, K. G., Heinig, M. J., Nommsen, L. A., et al. (1992). Growth of breast-fed and formula-fed infants from 0 to 18 months of age: The DARLING study. *Pediatrics, 89*, 1035–1041.

Faden, R. R., & Gielsen, A. (1986). Contemporary breast-feeding patterns: Focus on disadvantaged women. *Clinical Nutrition, 5*, 200–209.

Fallot, M. E., Boyd III, J. L., & Oski, F. A. (1980). Breast-feeding reduces incidence of hospital admissions for infection in infants. *Pediatrics, 65*, 1121–1124.

Finberg, L. (1987). Nutrition. In A. Rudolph (Ed.), *Pediatrics* (18th ed.). Norwalk, CT: Appleton & Lange.

Ford, K., & Labbok, M. (1990). Who is breast feeding? Implications of associated social and biomedical variables for research on the consequences of method of infant feeding. *American Journal of Clinical Nutrition, 52*, 451–456.

Frank, D. A., Wirtz, S. J., Sorenson, J. R., & Heeren, T. (1987). Commercial discharge packs and breast-feeding counseling: Effects on infant feeding practices in a randomized trial. *Pediatrics,*.

Freed, G. L., Landers, S., & Schanler, R. J. (1991). A practical guide to successful breast-feeding management. *American Journal of Diseases of Children, 145*, 917–921.

Greene, G. W., Smiciklas-Wright, H., Scholl, T. O., & Karp, R. J. (1988). Post partum weight change: How much of the weight gained in pregnancy will be lost after delivery? *Obstetrics and Gynecology, 71*, 701–707.

Kistin, N., Benton, D., Rao, S., & Sullivan, M. (1990). Breast-feeding rates among black urban low-income women: Effect of prenatal education. *Pediatrics, 86*, 741–746.

Klaus, M. H., & Kennell, J. H. (1976). *Maternal-infant bonding*. St. Louis: Mosby.

Kurinij, N., Shiono, P. H., & Rhoads, G. G. (1988). Breast-feeding: Incidence and duration in black and white women. *Pediatrics, 81*, 365–371.

Lawrence, R. A. (1989). *Breastfeeding: A guide for the medical profession*. St. Louis: Mosby.

Martinez, G. A., & Krieger, F. W. (1985). 1984 milk-feeding patterns in the United States. *Pediatrics, 76*, 1004–1008.

Meyer, H. F. (1966). Breast-feeding in the United States: Report of a 1966 national survey with comparable 1946 and 1956 data. *Clinical Pediatrics, 7*, 708–715.

Morley, R., Cole, T. J., Powell, R., & Lucas, A. (1988). Mother's choice to provide breast milk and developmental outcome. *Archives of Diseases of Children, 63*, 1382–1385.

Nelson, S. E., Ziegler, E. E., Copeland, A. M., et al. (1988). Lack of adverse reactions to iron-fortified formula. *Pediatrics, 81*, 360–364.

Perez, A., Vela, P., Masnick, G., & Potter, R. (1972). First ovulation after childbirth: The effect of breast-feeding. *American Journal of Obstetrics and Gynecology, 114*, 1041–1047.

Ryan, A. S., Rush, D., Krieger, F. W., & Lewandowski, G. E. (1991). Recent declines in breast-feeding in the United States, 1984 through 1989. *Pediatrics, 88*, 719–727.

Surgeon General. (1984). *Report of workshop on breastfeeding and human lactation*. Washington, DC (DHHS Public Health Service Publication No. HRS-D-MC-84–2, p. 20).

Tognetti, J., Hirschman, J. D., & McLaughlin, J. E. (1991). Decline in breastfeeding (Letter). *Pediatrics, 88*, 873–874.

Winikoff, B., Lauharan, V. H., Myers, D., & Stone, R. (1986). Dynamics of infant feeding: Mothers, professionals, and the institutional context in a large urban hospital. *Pediatrics, 77*, 357–365.

Worthington-Roberts, & Vermeesch, W. (1981). *Nutrition in pregnancy and lactation* (2nd ed., pp. 172–183). St. Louis: Mosby.

6

Nutritional Assessment of Disadvantaged Children

Darwin Deen, Jr., MD

The special concern of this chapter is to address the special needs of children growing up in the adverse circumstances to which we give the generic name "disadvantaged." The most dramatic form of undernutrition is protein-calorie malnutrition (PCM). Primary PCM is a rare occurrence in the United States, but secondary PCM is equivalent to nonorganic failure to thrive and is often caused by failure to nurture. PCM is now found as a common secondary effect of acquired immunodeficiency syndrome (AIDS), cancer, cystic fibrosis, and other chronic medical problems in childhood.

By tradition, techniques of nutritional assessment are divided into history, physical examination including anthropometric measurements and an estimation of body composition, and laboratory measurements.

HEALTH HISTORY

Many aspects of the routine medical, family, and social history have an impact on nutritional status including medical diagnosis, economic status of the family, and the parent's level of education. A chaotic social situation may be the first indication that a child's nutritional status needs further investigation (Karp, 1990). Thus, the first step in assessing nutritional status is to obtain a good health history to identify problems that may have a nutritional impact and thus dictate further evaluation or referral to a dietitian, and also to educate parents regarding normal nutrition.

"At-Risk" Concept in Nutritional Assessment

An "at-risk" concept should be used as a first step in any nutritional assessment (Jelliffe & Jelliffe, 1972). "At-risk" means the presence of "(a) biologic or environmental factors that predispose to disease. . . , and (b) easily recognizable early warning signs that malnutrition is impending" (p. 199).

Each and every child carries a set of risks that, if identified, establish the nature of the appropriate nutritional assessment. Recognizing factors that make the child at risk limits the number of false-positive tests that may result from unwarranted assessment.

Any of the following would make a child at risk for malnutrition: poverty, lack of social support, signs of child abuse or neglect, parent-child problems, lack of parental education or illiteracy, drug or alcohol abuse, teen pregnancy, chronic illness (or its treatment), and food cult behavior in the family.

To give some specific examples, children with overweight parents are at risk for obesity especially when they are from immigrant populations where fatness is preferred for children (Dietz, 1987). Similarly, assessment for iron deficiency is essential in disadvantaged children, but children from affluent families are no longer considered at risk (Dallman & Yip, 1989).

Dilemma of the Recommended Daily Allowances (RDAs)

RDAs were established to recommend a level of nutrient intake sufficient to keep healthy children and adults healthy. Although this may seem straightforward, critics point out that RDA makes policy based on current practice rather than nutritional science. An alternative position is that the RDA should recommend nutrient intakes so as to protect vulnerable populations such as children prone to iron deficiency (Herbert, 1987) or women with long-standing calcium deficiency (Avioli, 1989). It took the nutrition community 5 years of rancorous debate to complete the most recent edition of the RDA (Committee on Dietary Allowances, 1989).

As G. Beaton (1989) writes,

> We are suddenly faced with two completely different meanings: the traditional view that the purpose of the dietary standards report is to describe "nutrient requirements" and the growing view that the reports should offer prescriptive advice about a desirable pattern of dietary intake. These meanings are based not only on conventional concerns about nutrient deficiencies (which are rare in the United States) but on relationship of the diet-borne factors with chronic disease.

THE DIET HISTORY

A dietary assessment is performed to evaluate the child's diet with respect to quantity, quality, and variety of foods consumed. Answers to questions regarding the number of meals or snacks offered, approximate portion sizes, and the proportion of offered foods consumed help the physician get a general picture of the child's eating habits and dietary pattern.

Because patients may try to please the interviewer with their answers, the astute clinician will recognize what assumptions his or her patients are making about the questioner's attitude. Although open-ended questions are the rule for medical interviews, offering leading questions that clearly demonstrate what a healthy diet is may serve as an educational intervention. Thus, rather than asking the father of a 5-year-old if the child is drinking low-fat milk, it is more effective to ask whether the family is using low-fat milk and, if so, does that include this child. The message must be "patient specific" (low-fat dairy products are not appropriate for children under 2 years of age or most children requiring extra calories).

Some limitations in the reliability of the diet history are listed in Table 6.1 (Eck, Klesges, & Hanson, 1989). A food inventory technique developed by Kurt Lewin (1943) may provide special insight into the food habits of the very poor family (Karp, Snyder, Fairorth, et al., 1984).

One way of improving the accuracy of dietary information is by requesting that the family keep a food record for a certain number of days, especially when children have been labeled as "poor eaters" but are growing normally. It is helpful in reassuring parents to have formal documentation of quantities of food consumed. This methodology, although difficult to comply with, avoids the problems of memory and helps to focus attention on the pattern of meals/snacks, and the vari-

TABLE 6.1 Limitations in Reliability of Diet History

1. Parents may not accurately remember what the child has eaten.
2. Children's reliability depends upon their age, familiarity with the foods presented, how much they liked the food, and the setting for the meal.
3. Children frequently don't eat all of what they are offered, so that while questions regarding what is offered help to establish variety, they may not reflect adequacy of dietary intake.
4. Food is often consumed away from parental observation, e.g., at school or day care.

ety of foods offered and consumed. Quality of the diet can then be assessed by the number of fruits and vegetable servings provided; the amount and type of dairy products; the amount of foods of lower nutritional value (so-called junk food); and the frequency of use of meat, alternative protein sources, and whole grains.

NUTRITIONAL ASPECTS OF THE PHYSICAL EXAMINATION AND ANTHROPOMETRY

Examination

The importance of the clinician's overall impression of the patient cannot be over stressed (Baker et al., 1982). Chronic malnutrition not only produces growth failure and wasting, but also causes notable changes in hair, skin and oral mucosa, as well as behavioral abnormalities, such as psychomotor retardation and failure of normal interaction with caregivers and the outside world. Specific signs of deficiencies are shown in Table 6.2.

Anthropometry

For the pediatric population, anthropometry is probably the best tool for identifying nutritional problems, whether undernutrition (growth failure) or overnutrition (obesity). Anthropometric measurements were developed to assist in screening many people in field surveys. Their use in an office setting with an individual patient is often of benefit only if the measures are repeated serially so that data can be compared with previous measures in the same patient (Scholl, Cravioto, deLicardie, & Johnston, 1983). Discussion of the "height-age," "weight-age," and "ideal weight for actual height" is deferred to chapter 7, which discusses the growth of disadvantaged children.

The clinician who wishes to follow a patient's skin-fold measure-

TABLE 6.2 Specific Signs of Malnutrition

During the physical examination the areas most likely to show the effects of malnutrition are:

1. Hair—lack of normal pigmentation or luster, or easy pluckability.
2. Skin—dry, rough skin, petechiae, ecchymoses, or perifollicular hemorrhages.
3. Eyes—pale conjunctive, Bitot's spot or dull, dry conjunctiva (xerosis) or keratosis.
4. Lips, tongue and gums—cracked, fissured or pale lips, red, swollen tongue with loss of normal papillae, hemorrhages between the teeth.
5. Subcutaneous fat and musculoskeletal—wasting or obesity, bowed legs, epiphyseal enlargement and parietal bone enlargement.
6. Behavior—apathy, irritability, or other behavioral abnormalities.

ments must practice using calipers (the Lange or Harpenden) to ensure reliable results. Although easy to perform, skin-fold measurements are subject to greater error than height and weight, and must therefore be interpreted with caution. Interobserver variability is great, so one designated staff member should consistently perform these measures. Because normal ranges of skin-fold thickness vary with age, standards must be consulted (Frisancho, 1981).

Skin folds can be measured at a variety of sites. The one most frequently used is the triceps skin fold measured at the midpoint between the acromion and the olecranon process. Subscapular, biceps, and supraileac skin folds are often measured, and the sum of these four measurements may be used to calculate body fat.

Body Composition Estimations

From a nutritional standpoint, body mass may be considered to contain separate skeletal mass, adipose tissue, and protein compartments, with protein usually divided into skeletal muscle and visceral proteins (including visceral organs, serum proteins, and immunological proteins). Fomon and coworkers (1982) have published tables of body composition for reference children.

Patients with low weight-for-height, chronic diseases that affect growth, or problems with nutrient intake or use should have further assessment to determine which body compartments have been affected. The ratio of arm muscle circumference to head circumference has been used as a measure of chronic undernutrition (Sasanow, Georgieff, & Periera, 1986). Although obesity has been defined as being above the 90th percentile of the weight/height ratio, this method identifies "overweight," not "overfat." Dietz (1987) suggests that obesity be defined as a triceps skin fold greater than the 85th percentile.

Another method for estimating body fat is an elevated waist-to-hip ratio (Simopoulis). In adults, a ratio of more than one has been shown to increase cardiovascular disease risk. This needs further study in pediatric patients, particularly adolescents. Folsom, Burke, Ballew, et al. (1989) have recently shown that percent body fat and waist-to-hip ratio predicted cardiovascular disease risk factors in young adults. The body mass index (weight/height squared) may be helpful in defining "overfat" also.

Laboratory Evaluation

The specific tests used in laboratory assessment are deferred to the appropriate chapters. There are, however, some newer concepts in nutritional assessment to be considered.

As pointed out by Solomons (1981) in a recent review of the subject, functional measures of nutritional status, although not widely available, offer the possibility of monitoring the pathophysiological process created by nutrient deficiencies. Examples include measures of delayed hypersensitivity reactions as a marker of protein-calorie or zinc deficiency, dark adaptation vision tests as markers of vitamin A nutriture, and hand-grip strength as a marker of muscle function.

Malnutrition is a dynamic process, which begins in a healthy individual and progresses through periods of reduced nutrient intake or increased nutrient need. This causes tissue stores to decrease, followed by development of deficits in biochemical parameters that precede any clinical manifestation or physical abnormality. Functional indices offer the opportunity to detect marginal changes in nutritional status before the development of overt signs or symptoms.

The functional parameter most familiar to physicians is the monitoring of immune status via intradermal skin testing. Total lymphocyte count is also used as a measure of nutritional status and reflects the function of the reticuloendothelial system, as lymphopenia has serious consequences for host resistance.

Although functional measures of the immune system are not nutrient specific, they are able to provide a global assessment of nutritional status (e.g., growth is the ultimate functional test). Webb, Newman, Taylor, and Keogh (1989) recently studied hand-grip strength in adolescents and adults, and showed that postoperative complications were greater in those with less than 85% of predicted age standardized grip strength. The advantage of this technique is that it may allow us to detect changes in function that result from biochemical alterations but that precede the morphological changes measured by muscle circumference (Heymsfeld, 1982).

Although these methodologies are improving the ability of pediatric nutrition support specialists to assess body compartments accurately, some of them will be of use only in research settings. The techniques available to the general pediatrician continue to be a carefully taken history, physical examination, including anthropometrics, and the judicious use of the laboratory.

SUMMARY

This chapter has focused on the process for nutrition assessment available to the primary care clinician with a special emphasis on disadvantaged children. There is, in this setting, no substitute for a careful evaluation of the family, the child, the social setting in which they live, and the relationships among them.

Problems of undernutrition or overnutrition should be addressed on an ongoing basis. The participation of a dietitian on the health care team is essential. This is the best way to ensure continuous attention to the nutritional needs of disadvantaged children. The physician's role is to identify risks, begin a search for a diagnosis, initiate the referral process, and ensure compliance with dietary recommendations by reinforcing the information transmitted by the nutritionist at subsequent encounters with the patient. Team-delivered care is the preferred method of treatment for the nutritional problems of disadvantaged children. Health providers who have an understanding of the process of nutritional assessment will be better equipped to communicate with their registered dietitian colleagues and to integrate them into the care of patients and families to promote their patients' health better.

REFERENCES

Avioli, L. V. (1989). Calcium and phosphorus. In M. E. Shils, & V. Young (Eds.), *Modern nutrition in health and disease* (6th ed., pp. 142–158). Philadelphia: Lea and Febiger.

Baker, J. P., Detsky, A. S., Wesson, D. E., Wolman, S. L., Stewart, S., Whitewell, J., Langer, B., & Jeejeeboy, K. N. (1982). Nutritional assessment: A comparison of clinical judgment and objective measurements. *New England Journal of Medicine, 306*, 969–972.

Beaton, G. H. (1989). Criteria of an adequate diet. In M. E. Shils, & V. Young (Eds.), *Modern nutrition in health and disease* (6th ed., pp. 649–665). Philadelphia: Lea and Febiger.

Committee on Dietary Allowances, Food and Nutrition Board. (1989). Recommended Daily Allowances (10th rev. ed.). Washington, DC: National Academy of Sciences.

Dallman, P. R., & Yip, R. (1989). Changing characteristics of childhood anemia. *Journal of Pediatrics, 114*, 161–164.

Dietz, W. H. (1987). Child obesity. In R. J. Wurtman, & J. J. Wurtman (Eds.), Human obesity. *Annals of the New York Academy of Sciences, 499*, 47–54.

Eck, L. H., Klesges, R. C., & Hanson, C. L. (1989). Recall of a child's intake from one meal: Are parents accurate? *Journal of the American Dietetic Association, 89*, 784–789.

Fomon, S. J., Hasche, F., Ziegler, E. E., & Nelson, S. E. (1982). Body composition of reference children from birth to age 10 years. *American Journal of Clinical Nutrition, 35*, 1169–1175.

Folsom, A. R., Burke, G. L., Ballew, C., et al. (1989). Relation of body fatness and its distribution to cardiovascular risk factors in young blacks and whites. *American Journal of Epidemiology, 130*, 911–924.

Frisancho, A. R. (1981). New norms of upper limb fat and muscle area for assessment of nutritional status. *American Journal of Clinical Nutrition, 34*, 2540–2545.

Georgieff, M. K., Sasanow, S. R., Mammel, M. C., & Pereira, G. (1986). Mid-arm/head circumference ratios for identification of symptomatic LGA, AGA and SGA newborn infants. *Journal of Pediatrics, 109*, 316–321.

Herbert, V. (1987). Recommended daily intakes (RDI) of iron in humans. *American Journal of Clinical Nutrition, 45*, 679–686.

Heymsfield, S. B., Steven, V., Noel, R., McManus, C., Smith, J., & Nixon, D. (1982). Biochemical composition of muscle in normal and semi-starved human subjects: Relevance to anthropometric measurements. *American Journal of Clinical Nutrition, 36*, 131–142.

Jelliffe, D. B., & Jelliffe, E. F. P. (1972). The "at-risk" concept and young child nutrition programs (practices and principles). *Journal of Tropical Pediatrics, 18*, 199–201.

Karp, R. (1990). Malnutrition in the cycle of poverty. *Pediatric Annals, 19*, 265–275.

Karp, R. J., Snyder, E., Fairorth, J. W., et al. (1984). Parental behavior and the availability of foods among undernourished inner city school children. *Journal of Family Practice, 18*, 731.

Lewin, K. (1943). Forces behind food habits and methods of change. In The problem of changing food habits (Publication No. 108). Washington, DC.

Sasanow, S. R., Georgieff, M. K., Periera, G. R. (1986). Mid-arm circumference and mid-arm/head circumference ratios: standard curves for anthropometric assessment of neonatal nutritional status. *Journal of Pediatrics, 109*, 311–315.

Scholl, T. O., Cravioto, J., deLicardie, E., & Johnston, F. E. (1983). The utility of cross-sectional measurements of weight and length for age in screening for growth failure (chronic malnutrition) and clinically severe protein-energy malnutrition. *Acta Pediatrica Scandinavica, 72*, 867–872.

Solomons, N. W. (1981). Assessment of nutritional status: functional indicators of pediatric nutriture. *Pediatic Clinics of North America, 32*, 319–334.

Webb, A. R., Newman, L. A., Taylor, M., & Keogh, J. B. (1989). Hand grip dynanometry as a predictor of postoperative complications reappraisal using age standardized grip strengths. *Journal of Parenteral and Enteral Nutrition, 13*, 30–33.

7

Growth of Disadvantaged Children

Robert J. Karp, MD

Until recently, short stature in a population has been ascribed to "racial characteristics," that is, the growth of parents influencing the growth of their children. It was thought that members of different racial groups have different potentials for growth. As the 1962 edition of *Pediatrics* (edited by Holt, McIntosh, and Barnett) states, "It is certainly true that there are tall and short races and nations, The question may well be asked, however, whether postnatal influences, such as better nutrition and less illness, do not seriously obscure that this difference is hereditary" (p. 4).

But, as discussed in chapter 1, subsequent observations with large population groups (the older view may be correct for small tribes such as the Bantu) suggest that a reversal of concern should be made in the clinical diagnoses of short stature. A more appropriate statement, especially when evaluating a disadvantaged child, would be "familial differences in growth potential may obscure the conclusion that observed differences in growth are caused by poor nutrition, indifferent parenting, or by illness." (See Birch & Gussow, 1970.)

In this chapter we follow the growth of a child, noting parental (genetic) influences on growth as well as those occurring in utero and during early life. Methods for assessing nutritional status and for monitoring the effectiveness of therapy will be provided. Do the disadvantages listed earlier affect growth? How do we assess for growth retardation? How important is the stature of the parents? Can we determine when parents are effective? And, how do we treat the growth-retarded disadvantaged child?

ARE DISADVANTAGED CHILDREN SHORT?

"The dimensions of poverty," writes Stanley Garn, "are spelled out in the growth of children" (1975). In the United States, recognition that disadvantage existed at all had to precede a recognition that this disadvantage has effects on children, growth failure included. As discussed in the introduction to this book, in two large national surveys, The Ten State Nutritional Survey (Department of Health, Education and Welfare, 1972) and The Pre-School Nutrition Survey (Owen, Kram, Garry, et al., 1974), presumed undernutrition, shown by the prevalence of growth retardation and nutritional anemia, was more common among the poor, less-educated segment of the population. These studies considered children en masse and have been criticized, to play on a popular aphorism, for describing all "forest and no trees." For the purpose of this text, it is important to consider studies within poor communities where the heterogeneous nature of poverty is considered. In these communities all families are poor; some families are more likely to have the nutritional problems associated with poverty than others. Here we can look at the trees within the forest.

Three such communities were described in chapter 1. In a fourth example from the urban United States, Scholl, Karp, Theophano, and Decker (1987) have shown that white children in a poor urban community have an excessive prevalence of undernutrition as compared with black and Hispanic children. In this community, little if any undernutrition was found among the general population of black preschool and early school-age children. When, however, the same urban community studied by Scholl and colleagues was considered in the context of an important risk factor for growth retardation, child abuse, diminution in growth was found among black and Hispanic children (Karp, Scholl, Decker, & Ebert, 1989). And 10% of the white children attending several of the schools in this community showed a constellation of signs associated with FAS (Marino, Scholl, Karp, et al., 1987).

The data from these studies reinforce an image of poor communities as being heterogeneous. Disadvantage in the home experience or the prenatal environment is of more consequence than the disadvantage of poverty alone. The implication of these studies, taken as a whole, is that if all members of a society had similar advantage with respect to food, water supply, health care, and nurturing, they would exhibit growth similar to that of the most privileged sectors of society.

ASSESSMENT OF GROWTH

The Growth Curve

These are available with adjustments for age and sex from Ross Laboratories (Columbus, OH). Children must have measurements of growth accurately measured and plotted over a period. There are three reasons for this.

First, single measurements taken at a mass screening are useful for the assessment of the nutritional status of the community only (Scholl, Johnston, Cravioto, & deLicardie, 1983). A reduction in measurements means little about the nutritional status of any one child. Second, chronic malnutrition leads to stunting of linear growth (Waterlow, 1976). Unless there is concomitant acute malnutrition with wasting, the child will appear to be younger than his or her chronological age. *It is only by plotting measurements that undernutrition will be identified* (*Lancet*, editorial, 1990).

Finally, calculation of the "height age," "weight age," and "ideal weight for actual height" from the growth curves is necessary in the treatment of the affected children (see case study later in this chapter) (Goldbloom, 1987).

Classification Systems

There are three systems currently used to assess the quality of growth. These are the Gomez (Jelliffe, 1966), the Waterlow (1976), and the McLaren and Reed (Goldbloom, 1987) scores. The Gomez is a weight-for-age system that is used in developing countries though not in the United States.

The Waterlow system considers weight for age and weight for length (or height)—first separately and then together as shown in Table 7.1. "Wasting" (decreased weight for length) is associated with acute malnutrition and is distinguished from stunting (decreased length or height for age) as is seen with chronic malnutrition.

The Waterlow system is used to present data from population studies. As Martorell has shown, wasted or stunted children are at greater risk from death from infection than children with neither wasting nor stunting (1985). With respect to intellectual development, Powell and

TABLE 7.1 Classification and Definition of Protein-Energy Malnutrition

		length or height for age	
		'OK'	<5th%
weight for length or height	'OK'	normal	stunting (chronic p-c.m)
	<5th%	wasting (acute p-c.m)	both acute & chronic p-c.m

From Waterlow, 1976.

Grantham-McGregor (1985) have shown stunted children to suffer greater developmental deficit than wasted children. In a subsequent study Simeon and Grantham-McGregor (1989) showed deleterious effects on learning ability among children who had a past history of either wasting or stunting.

The third system, of McLaren and Read, best describes the pathophysiology of growth retardation (Goldbloom, 1987). The ratio of actual weight to ideal weight for actual height is calculated and used to determine the degree of protein-energy malnutrition and to plan therapy.

Arm Anthropometry

Under special circumstances it may be necessary to measure the circumference of the arm and the triceps fat fold as these will be influenced by food intake. The techniques are described by Jelliffe (1966) and Frisancho (1974), who provides tables for assessment.

PARENTS

How Did They Grow?

There are two types of genetic short stature. In "familial short stature," one or both of the parents are short, and the child inherits "short genes." It is common within population groups for people who are alike to marry one another; for two short parents or for two tall ones, adjustment for midparental height may show whether the actual height is appropriate for the genetic potential. These tables are available from Ross Laboratories. With one tall and one short parent, the adjustment for midparental height is less helpful.

The other form of genetic short stature is referred to as "constitutional." Here the child grows at the lower percentiles for a longer time and ultimately achieves a height close to, or even above, average. The parents may give a similar history of growth, and the mother often has had menarche at a late age.

How Do They Parent?

Careful history and observation must be used to identify children who fail to grow because of emotional deprivation (Berwick, 1980; Goldbloom, 1987). These will be the overwhelming majority of growth-retarded children presenting to an ambulatory care setting in a disadvantaged community. It is possible to make a diagnosis of nonorganic failure to thrive (NOFTT) from historical evidence gathered from the home environment. The first consideration is whether there are structural problems in the home that are overwhelming the caretakers (Berwick, 1980). To be considered are (a) too many children, too close in age; (b) a young mother with an inadequate support system; (c) evidence of drug or alcohol abuse; (d) overcrowding or otherwise unhealthy conditions such as lack of clean water or refrigeration, and too little available nutritious food as are associated with homelessness.

It is necessary to observe the mother-child interaction for evidence of poor parenting. The behavior of the child may suggest psychosocial deprivation. These children seem withdrawn from their environment, and are unlikely to smile or otherwise reach out to people or objects in their environment; they lack the curiosity that is so delightful in contented infants. Sometimes they exhibit socially inappropriate behavior such as head banging or rocking obsessively. Children who fail to grow because of illness rarely behave in this way.

Often clerks in the clinic are the first to observe problems in parent-child interactions that are hidden from the professional staff. They should be encouraged to share their observations, in private, with the health care providers.

Although it is essential to keep eyes, ears, and feelings open, there are objective measures to help in the assessment of appropriate behavior. Two scales used are the Polansky Child Level of Living Scale (1978) and the Caldwell HOME inventory (Casey, 1984). A part of the Polansky scale is shown as Table 7.2. Information related to nutrition can be used to assess both nutritional adequacy and parenting (Karp, Snyder, Fairorth, et al., 1984).

In three studies of undernourished children, Pollitt (1975), Casey, Bradley, and Wortham (1984); and Karp et al. (1984) showed a correla-

TABLE 7.2 Polansky Child Level of Living Scale (1978)

NOTE: Fill out 1 to 4 without additional questions

1. The parent provides at least one meal each day consisting of two courses (either meat and vegetable or two vegetables) _____
2. The parent plans for variety in foods _____
3. The parent plans meals with courses that go together _____
4. The child is offered meals at fixed times each day _____

ASK, "Are you happy with the foods _____ eats?"
This gives the parent a chance to express concern.
You ask, "Why?" and she/he can make statement for questions 5 and 6.

5. The parent expresses concern about feeding the child a balanced diet _____
6. The parent mentions that she makes an effort to get the child to eat foods not preferred because they are important for good nutrition _____

ASK, "What did _____ have at _____ (name last holiday)?"

7. The parent plans special meals for special occasions _____
8. (for older children) The parent encourages the child to wash hands before meals _____

tion between parenting, as measured by these scales, and nutritional status.

PRENATAL LIFE OF THE CHILD

Bacon Chow speculated, some 30 years ago, that the fetus seemed to make a judgment as to what kind of world he or she would inhabit based on the availability of nutrients in utero (Adair & Pollitt, 1985). Current research gives some validity to this theory. In a review of the Tennessee WIC program, Binken, Yip, Fleshood, & Trowbridge (1988) note, "Infants with lower birth weights were likely to remain shorter and lighter throughout childhood, especially those who were intrauterine growth retarded rather than premature." Early disadvantage, taken in its broadest meaning, may result in the birth of a child programed to be small. Though catch-up in growth and development is the common sequel to intrauterine growth retardation, when a child born to a disadvantaged mother continues to live in a disadvantaged environment, catch-up is less likely (Warshaw, 1986) as the potential for correction seems to be set during the first 18 months of life (Martorell, 1985).

There is a substantial literature on nutrition in prenatal life, beginning with conception. Significant reductions in one or more micronutrient levels can be found with cigarette smoking, adolescent pregnancy, alcohol consumption, use of oral contraceptives, and among the poor in general. The effects of micronutrient deficiencies (specifically folic acid) in the mother at conception on the growth of the developing human fetus have been subject to much discussion that is beyond the scope of this chapter (see Mulinare, Cordero, Erikson, & Berry, 1988).

Later in pregnancy, caloric intake of the mother becomes a major influence on the growth of the fetus. Intrauterine growth retardation caused by nutritional deprivation results in a child who is small in weight for gestational age (SGA). The reductions in growth will occur in arm circumference, weight, length, and head circumference in that order (Stein, Susser, Marolla, & Saenger, 1975). Sasanow, Georgieff, and Periera (1986) have used this phenomenon to develop arm circumference (most affected) to head circumference (least affected) ratio curves to distinguish between nutritionally induced SGA and prematurity induced appropriateness of weight for gestational age (AGA). Note that a reduction in head circumference below expected levels suggests *in utero* exposure to alcohol (see chapter 10).

HEALTH OF CHILD

Of most importance organic and nonorganic (deprivation) growth failure are not mutually exclusive phenomenon. Growth is mediated by activities within all organ systems in the body. A family with limited resources may respond in ways to disease in a child to create an inhospitable environment for that child. Widdowson has shown growth failure with caloric intake she thought to be adequate (1951). Powell and colleagues have provided evidence that an impairment in growth hormone secretion occurs with emotional deprivation (1967). The accepted view, however, is that growth failure, in the absence of a hypermetabolic state, is always associated with a reduced caloric intake (Goldbloom, 1987; *Lancet*, editorial, 1990). Thus, assessment begins with a careful review of the diet.

Nutritional Status Effects Growth

Both iron and zinc deficiencies are associated with growth retardation. Studies by Prasad and Halsted in Iran and Egypt showed a syndrome of poor growth, sexual immaturity, and zinc deficiency in communities where the diet was high in unrefined wheat flour (Prasad, Halsted, & Nadimi, 1961). Though the oral intake of zinc as well as iron was, in theory, sufficient to provide adequate micronutrients, the presence of excessive phytates and fibers prevented absorbtion. These children responded to zinc supplementation with an increase in caloric intake and with growth.

In 1972, Hamidge, Hamidge, Jacobs, et al. observed an association with reduced growth and anorexia among children in a poor community in Denver, Colorado. In this first set of studies, zinc supplementation resulted in an increase in linear growth, suggesting a direct effect on intermediary zinc metabolism rather than on appetite. In a second set of studies (Walravens, Hamidge, & Koepfer, 1988), the effect was an increase both in caloric intake and weight, suggesting appetite effects. A more recent study by Gibson, Vanderkooy, MacDonald, et al. (1989), in southern Ontario, provided results similar to those in the first Denver study.

It cannot be determined from these studies how zinc deficiency affects growth. Is there hypoguesia and decreased appetite from the effect on taste perception? It is more likely that the catch-up growth found is mediated through the requirement of zinc for growth, but perhaps there is a synergism of the two effects.

An additional variable is alcohol consumption and its effect on zinc metabolism and growth. Alcohol exposure in utero is associated with an embryopathy of FAS, which includes (as will be discussed in chapter 10) growth retardation. Taste perception of FAS children has not been studied, but, more important, FAS should be considered in subsequent studies of growth-retarded children.

For much of the early era of bottle-feeding, it was a common finding to have a milk-fed, overfed, and thus overweight, infant who was iron deficient. An unrecognized associated finding was growth retardation (Judisch, Naiman, & Oski, 1966). Karp et al. (1984) showed that iron deficiency and mild growth retardation among early school-age children were associated with increased intake of foods of low nutrient density (so-called junk food) as part of a convenience food–dependant diet. These studies suggest that aberrations in diet, including excess consumption of cow's milk, high-fiber intake, and a dependence on convenience foods among the poor, may result in iron deficiency and growth retardation.

Case Study Showing Treatment

Travis B. was born at 38 weeks' gestation to a cocaine-using mother who had poor prenatal care. Travis did poorly at home, and his failure to thrive required social as well as nutritional intervention. He was 8 months of age with a length of 65 cm (26.5 inches) and a weight of 5.8 kg (12.8 pounds) when he presented to the Pediatric Resource Center of Kings County Hospital. This length gave him a length age of 4.5 months. At 4.5 months of age, mean body weight is 7.0 kg, thus his "actual weight as percent of ideal weight for actual height" is 5.8/7.0 = 0.83 suggesting moderate malnutrition (Goldbloom, 1987). Travis, like many undernourished infants was also iron deficient. (See figure 7.1.)

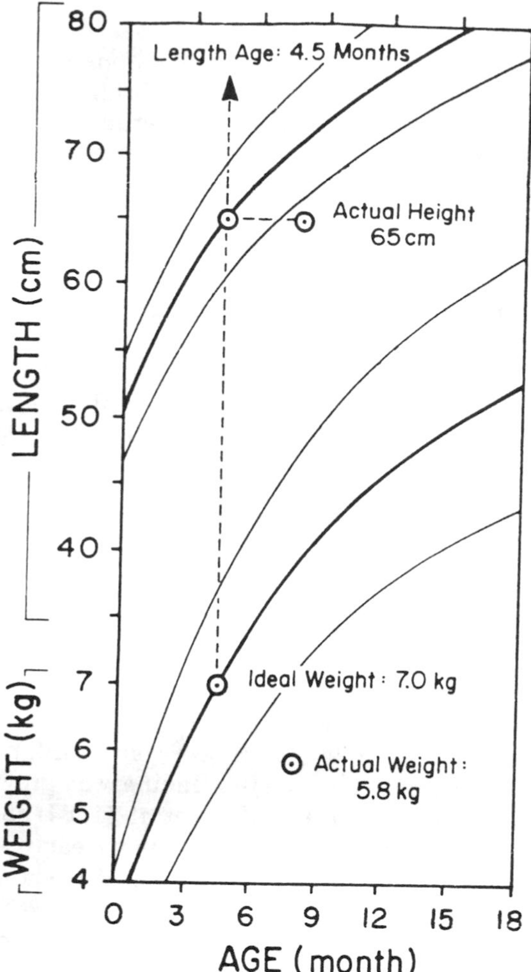

FIGURE 7.1 Height and weight for Travis.

Calculation for Travis: To calculate "actual weight as a percentage of ideal weight for actual height or length:" (McLaren & Reed, 1975).

1. Plot actual height or length for age and sex.
2. Draw a horizontal line to the 50th percentile.
3. Draw a vertical line to indicate the "height or length age."
4. Continue the vertical line to the 50th percentile on the weight for age curve.
5. Draw a horizontal line to show the "ideal weight for actual height or length."
6. Form the fraction "actual weight/ideal weight for actual height or length."
7. Determine nutritional status according to the standards below:

Degree of protein-energy malnutrition	Weight as percentage of ideal weight for actual height or length
Normal	90–110
Mild	85–90
Moderate	75–85
Severe	<75

Ashworth and Millward (1986) have shown that wasted children will not achieve catch-up growth without extra calories. They must not be fed a "prudent" diet with only 30% of calories from fat. A caloric supplement of 50% above that which would be provided for a well-nourished child of the same weight is suggested. Careful and frequent follow-up must be maintained. Haste in establishing adequate caloric intake is not advised, however, in that this amount of food may be unacceptable to a starving child if provided immediately. A 3- to 5-day period of accelerated feedings is suggested.

Travis needed sufficient energy for a healthy child of 9 kg or 900 calories plus a boost of 300 to 400 calories for growth. Travis was given 18 mg of ferrous sulfate (3 mg/kg) to be continued for 3 months. An aunt took over the care of Travis and subsequently adopted him.

Health professionals may find it difficult to promote diets high in fat and cholesterol even when they are essential. These are, in fact, the desired foods for a child such as Travis at this point in his life. Subsequent to the refeeding, a usual infant diet, as described in chapter 5 will be resumed.

Catch-up in the weight age for the wasted child should begin almost immediately and will bring the child out of the acute phase of malnutrition. A 3-month period may be needed before catch-up in height-age can be seen. For children in good foster care or where the underlying problem of nurturing in the family is corrected, there is a tendency at this point in therapy for the children to become overweight.

Do not lose these children and their families in follow-up. This is a sign of drifting away from health care. Travis failed to grow again at one year of age when he developed reactive airway disease, but his aunt was cooperative in the evaluation and therapy, and Travis recovered again. Most important, Travis is a developmentally normal child. This is the best outcome.

ACKNOWLEDGMENT

The help of Jane Federman, MD, in the preparation of this chapter is greatly appreciated.

REFERENCES

Adair, L. S., & Pollitt, E. (1985). Outcome of nutritional supplementation: a comprehensive review of the Bacon Chow study. *American Journal of Clinical Nutrition, 41*, 948–978.

Ashworth, A., & Millward, D. J. (1986). Catch-up growth in children. *Nutrition Reviews, 44*, 157–163.

Berwick, D. M. (1980). Nonorganic Failure to Thrive. *Pediatrics in Review, 1*, 265–270.

Binkin, N. J., Yip, R., Fleshood, L., & Trowbridge, F. L. (1988). Birth weight and childhood growth. *Pediatrics, 82*, 828–834.

Birch, H. G., Gussow, J. D. (1970). *Disadvantaged children: Health, nutrition, and school failure* (chapter 5). New York: Harcourt Brace & World; Grune & Stratton.

Casey, P. H., Bradley, R., & Wortham, B. (1984). Social and nonsocial home environments of infants with non-organic failure to thrive. *Pediatrics, 73*, 348.

Frisancho, A. R. (1974). Triceps skinfold and upper arm muscle size norms for assessment of nutritional status. *American Journal of Clinical Nutrition, 27*, 1052–1058.

Garn, S. M., & Clark, D. C. (1975). Nutrition, growth, development and malnutrition: Findings from the 10-State Nutrition Survey of 1968–70. *Pediatrics, 56*, 306–319.

Gibson, R. S., Vanderkooy, P. D. S., MacDonald, A. C., et al. (1989). A growth-limiting, mild zinc deficiency in some southern Ontario boys with low height percentiles. *American Journal of Clinical Nutrition, 49*, 1266–1273.

Goldbloom, R. B. (1987). Growth failure in infancy. *Pediatrics in Review, 9*, 57–61.

Hamidge, K. M., Hamidge, C., Jacobs, M., et al. (1972). Low levels of zinc in hair, anorexia, poor growth and hypoguesia in children. *Pediatric Research, 6*, 868–874.

Holt, L. E., Jr., McIntosh, R., & Barnett, H. (1962). *Pediatrics* (13th ed., pp. 1–41). New York: Appleton-Century Crofts.

Jelliffe, D. B. (1966). *The assessment of nutritional status in the community* (Monograph Series No. 53). Geneva, Switzerland: World Health Organization.

Judisch, J. M., Naiman, J. L., & Oski, F. A. (1966). The fallacy of the fat iron-deficient child. *Pediatrics, 37*, 987–990.

Karp, R. J., Scholl, T. O., Decker, E., & Ebert, E. (1989). Growth of abused children contrasted with the non-abused in an urban poor community. *Clinics in Pediatrics, 28*, 317–320.

Karp, R., Snyder, E., Fairorth, J. W., et al. (1984). Parental behavior and the availability of foods among undernourished inner-city school children. *Journal of Family Practice, 18*, 731.

(1990). Failure to thrive revisited. [Editorial]. *Lancet, 336*, 662–663.

Marino, R. V., Scholl, T. O., Karp, R. J., et al. (1987). Minor physical anomalies and learning disability: What is the prenatal component? *Journal of the National Medical Association, 79*, 37–39.

Martorell, R. (1985). Child growth and nutrition: a discussion of its causes and relationship to health. In J. C. Waterlow, K. Blaxter, (Eds.), *Nutritional adaptation* (pp. 13–30). London: John Libbey.

Mulinare, J., Cordero, J. F., Erikson, J. D., & Berry, R. J. (1988). Periconceptual use of vitamins and the occurrence of neural tube deficits. *Journal of the American Medical Association, 260*, 3141–3145.

Owen, G. M., Kram, K. M., Garry, P. J., et al. (1974). A study of nutritional status of pre-school children in the United States, 1968–1970. *Pediatrics, 53*, 597–646.

Polansky, N., Chalmers, M. A., Buttonweiser, E., & Williams, I. (1978). Child Level of Living Scale: an urban view. *Child Welfare, 62*, 439.

Politt, E. (1975). Failure to thrive: Socioeconomic, dietary intake and mother-child interaction data. *Federation Proceedings, 34*, 1593.

Powell, C. A., & Grantham-McGregor, S. (1985). The ecology of nutritional status and development in young children in Kingston, Jamaica. *American Journal of Clinical Nutrition, 41*, 1322–1331.

Powell, G. F., Brasel, J. A., Raiti, S., & Blizzard, R. M. (1967). Emotional deprivation and growth retardation simulating idiopathic hypopituitarism: II. Endocrinologic evaluation of syndrome. *New England Journal of Medicine, 276*, 1279–1283.

Prasad, A. S., Halsted, J. A., & Nadimi, M. (1961). Syndrome of iron deficiency anemia, hepatosplenomegaly, hypogonadism, dwarfism and geophagia. *American Journal of Medicine, 31*, 532–546.

Sasanow, S. R., Georgieff, M. K., & Perera, G. R. (1986). Mid-arm circumference and midarm/head circumference ratios: standard curves for anthropometric assessment of neonatal nutritional status. *Journal of Pediatrics, 109*, 311–315.

Scholl, T. O., Karp, R. J., Theophano, J., & Decker, E. (1987). Ethnic differences in growth and nutritional status: a study of poor schoolchildren in southern New Jersey. *Public Health Reports, 102*, 278–283.

Scholl, T. O., Johnston, F. E., Cravioto, J., & deLicardie, E. R. (1983). The utility of cross-sectional measurements of weight and length for age in screening for growth failure and clinically severe protein energy malnutrition. *Acta Pediatrica Scandinavica, 72*, 867–870.

Simeon, D. T., &, Grantham-McGregor, S. (1989). Effects of missing breakfast on the cognitive function of school children of differing nutritional status. *American Journal of Clinical Nutrition, 49*, 646–653.

Stein, Z., Susser, M., Marolla, F., & Saenger, G. (1975). *Famine and human development: the Dutch hunger winter of 1944–45*. New York: Oxford University Press.

U.S. Department of Health, Education and Welfare, Health Services and Mental Health Administration. (1972). *The Ten-State Nutrition Survey, 1968, 1970*. (DHEW Publication No. [HSM] 72-8130 to 72-8134). Atlanta: Centers for Disease Control.

Walravens, P. A., Hamidge, K. M., & Koepfer, D. M. (1989). Zinc supplementation in infants with a nutritional pattern of failure to thrive: A double blind, controlled study. *Pediatrics, 83*, 532–538.

tion. In J. Bengoa & G. Beaton (Eds.), *Nutrition in preventive medicine* (pp. 530–555). Geneva, Switzerland: World Health Organization..

Widdowson, E. M. (1951). Mental contentment and physical growth. *Lancet, 1*, 1316–1318.

8

Iron Deficiency Among Disadvantaged Children

Betsy Lozoff, MD, and Robert J. Karp, MD

Iron deficiency anemia is among the most common nutritional deficiencies in the world. With peak prevalence in infancy, perhaps 25% of all babies are affected. Anemia is a late manifestation of iron deficiency. An even greater percentage of children of all ages shows the biochemical changes of iron lack that precede the development of iron deficiency anemia. It is during these early stages that prevention can occur.

This chapter considers recent evidence from research on central nervous system biochemistry in lower animals and from studies of human infants that iron deficiency adversely affects behavior by impairing cognitive function and producing noncognitive disturbances. This body of research, taken as a whole, provides increasingly persuasive arguments for intensifying efforts to prevent and treat iron deficiency anemia.

PREVALENCE

The prevalence of iron deficiency anemia in the United States is greatly influenced by poverty and lack of education (Ten State Nutrition Survey, 1971; Owen, Kram, Garry, et al., 1974). As shown in the introduction to this book, hemoglobin levels have been substantially lower among children from the lowest socioeconomic status group. Supporting these findings was a study in 1971 of children 9 to 36 months of age from a lower socioeconomic status section of New Haven, Connecticut. The mean hemoglobin (Hgb) was 11.1 g/dl with the 5th percentile for Hgb of 7.7 g/dl (Vazquez-Seoane et al., 1985). The iron status of U.S. children has improved substantially in recent years. The causes for this improvement will be discussed in the concluding section of this chapter.

CONSEQUENCES

Until recently it was often presumed that iron deficiency anemia had few deleterious effects unless severe enough to compromise cardiovascular function. However, in the past decade evidence that iron deficiency has important behavioral effects has accumulated steadily. The resulting picture of behavioral alterations owing to iron deficiency reflects the convergence of two independent but complementary investigational approaches: (a) studies of central nervous system biochemical changes, primarily in the laboratory animal; and (b) studies of behavior before and after iron treatment, primarily in the young human.

Other correlates of iron deficiency in childhood include proneness to pica with increased lead burden (Crosby, 1976; Lanzkowsky, 1959) and possible growth retardation (Judisch et al., 1966; Oski, 1984). These concerns are discussed elsewhere in the text. Studies among older children have detected changes in attentional processes and in oddity and discrimination learning, which seemed to improve with iron therapy (Lozoff, 1990), but few replicated results are available. Therefore, this review will focus on the major consequence of iron deficiency anemia among infants and indicate the ways in which iron deficiency may adversely effect behavior and learning potential, especially among the disadvantaged.

In animal studies it is possible to make certain that iron-deficient animals differ from controls only in their dietary iron intake; adequate intake of other nutrients can be controlled, and genetic endowment and rearing conditions can be made the same. However, in human populations, nutritional disorders are not uniformly distributed. They are more likely to occur in the context of poverty, environmental deprivation, and disadvantaged social conditions, all of which may adversely affect behavior and development (Lozoff, 1989, 1990).

Iron deficiency is most prevalent in the 6- to 24-month-old period, which coincides with the latter part of the brain growth spurt and

TABLE 8.1 Table Title To Come

IRON STATUS GROUP	(N)	Hemoglobic Level (g/dl)	Iron Measures (ferritin, EP, transferrin saturation)
Sufficient	(35)	≥12.0	all normal
Depleted	(38)	≥12.0	↓ ferritin
Deficient (no anemia)	(21)	≥12.0	↓ ferritin plus ↑ EP or ↓ saturation
Deficient (intermediate)	(45)	10.6-11.9	↓ ferritin plus ↑ EP or ↓ saturation
Deficient (Mild anemia)	(18)	10.1-10.5	↓ ferritin plus ↑ EP or ↓ saturation
Deficient (moderate anemia)	(34)	≤10.0	↓ ferritin plus ↑ EP or ↓ saturation

with the unfolding of fundamental mental and motor processes. Several recent studies have yielded a set of findings that has been reproducible in broad general outline, even though some of the specific results still await replication. Taken as a group, these studies have been designed to establish whether behavioral alterations are present among iron-deficient infants, and to address three further questions: (a) What is the degree of iron deficiency at which infant behavior is altered? (b) Does iron therapy produce rapid changes in behavior? (c) Does iron therapy completely correct these behavioral alterations?

At What Degree Does Iron Deficiency Affect Behavior?

The first question has been studied because iron deficiency occurs along a physiological continuum. Reductions in total body iron have been grouped into three stages of progressively increasing severity: (a) iron depletion, (b) iron deficiency without anemia, and (c) iron deficiency anemia. At what point in the continuum of iron deficiency is infant behavior adversely affected? A recent study in Costa Rica by Lozoff et al. (1987) enrolled in a single study a relatively large number of otherwise healthy infants with varied iron status. The sample consisted of 191 12- to 23-month-old infants divided into groups ranging from least to most iron-deficient as shown in Table 8.1.

In the study, the Bayley Scales of Infant Development (1969) were administered before and after 1 week and after 3 months of intramuscular or oral iron with appropriate placebo controls. Infants with moderate iron de-

erate iron deficiency anemia were found to have lower mental and motor test scores than the rest of the sample, and infants with mild anemia received lower motor scores but not mental scores. The mean mental test score of the moderately anemic infants was 8 points below that of infants with higher Hgb levels, and the mean motor score of the entire anemic group was 10 points below that of infants with Hgb > 10.5 g/dl. Infants with iron depletion or iron deficiency with intermediate or normal Hgb levels did not receive lower mental or motor developmental test scores.

The results of the Costa Rican project are noteworthy for several reasons. The study was community based, thus minimizing biases potentially involved in research with patient populations. Infants with all known risk factors for altered hematological or developmental status had been carefully excluded. Iron-deficient and iron-depleted conditions were confirmed by hematological response to iron therapy. Finally, an extensive set of background variables relating to birth, general nutritional status, lead level, family background, home environment, and parental IQ failed to reveal any factor other than iron deficiency anemia that might explain the findings.

Moreover, the findings were replicated in a recent study by Walter and associates in Chile (1989). Because of its prospective design, the new study by Walter et al. provides insight into the importance of chronicity and severity in iron deficiency anemia. Those infants who were anemic at both 9 and 12 months had significantly lower developmental test scores than those with anemia of less than 3 months' duration. Thus, research published to date supports the conclusion that iron deficiency severe enough to cause anemia is associated with impaired performance on mental development tests in infancy before treatment.

Are There Rapid Changes With Iron Treatment?

Until the last 2 or 3 years, most studies examining the behavioral effects of iron deficiency were designed to detect changes in developmental test performance within 5 to 11 days of starting iron therapy. Clinicians, in describing iron-deficient anemic babies as irritable, apathetic, and distractable, have commented that these characteristics seem to disappear within a few days of iron treatment (Lozoff & Brittenham, 1985), suggesting that the behavioral changes reflect altered central nervous system function rather than the correction of anemia. However, studies including a placebo condition found increases in scores regardless of the iron or placebo treatment the infants received, or their iron status before treatment (Lozoff, 1989, 1990). The results if the Bayley Scales are readministered after a short period, and they cannot be attributed to iron therapy (see chapters 2 and 3 for discussion of the implications of developmental testing).

Is There Complete Correction With Iron Therapy?

Although separating the effects of iron deficiency from those of anemia is important, a more pertinent question from a clinical perspective is whether or not iron therapy completely corrects any behavioral abnormalities, regardless of how soon changes might be detectable.

Until very recently, none of the infant studies could address this issue, because none included assessments after a course of iron therapy. The study in Costa Rica was specifically designed to examine the effects of a course of treatment commonly used in practice—3 months of oral iron therapy. All infants responded to treatment by attaining normal hemoglobin levels, but, as would be expected, some of them still showed biochemical evidence of iron deficiency, especially a high erythrocyte protoporphyrin (EP) level. On the basis of hematological response to iron therapy, infants who became iron sufficient by the conclusion of the study were distinguished from those who did not correct all evidence of iron deficiency. Though the improvement in motor scores was substantial and indicates a beneficial effect of treatment, a worrisome result is that most anemic infants did not show improvements with iron therapy.

These studies cannot determine whether the ill effects of iron deficiency anemia persist beyond infancy. The lower mental and motor test scores among many of the iron-deficient anemic infants might have responded to a more extended course of iron therapy. It is also possible that the deficits might persist even if laboratory evidence of iron deficiency had been entirely corrected in all the anemic infants. This outcome would indicate that iron deficiency anemia in infancy, perhaps of a particular severity or chronicity, has long-lasting ill effects. Alternatively, these differences might disappear spontaneously, especially because, as Sewell and colleagues note in chapter 3, Bayley scores in the second year of life are only moderately correlated with measures of cognitive function in childhood. However, the formerly anemic children in the Costa Rican and Chilean studies continued to show lower test scores when reevaluated at 5 to 5½ years of age. By contrast, Idjradinata and Pollitt (1993) found that intensive iron therapy (sufficient to replace iron stores) was associated with a reversal of developmental delays in formerly iron-deficient infants.

NUTRITIONAL ADAPTATION IN IRON DEFICIENCY

When a child has sufficient iron, the cells lining the surface of the small intestine have full ferritin content. Iron passing by does not en-

TABLE 8.2 Relationship Between Iron Absorption and Iron Status for Several Food Types

Iron Source	Approximate Absorption of Iron (%) Iron Sufficient	Iron Deficient
Ferrous Ascorbate	7	45
Hemoglobin	10	20
Ferritin	6	12
Wheat	4	6

Moore, 1968.

ter the cell and is passed in the stool. As Table 8.2 shows, iron absorption in the iron-sufficient person is low (about 10%) with all sources of iron. In the earliest stages of iron deficiency—iron depletion—the ferritin content of the endothelial cells decreases. Dietary iron from within the gastrointestinal tract then enters the cell more easily. In the next stage, iron deficiency without anemia, there is decreased circulating iron bound to transferrin. The transfer of iron from intracellular to circulation bound to transferrin is therefore facilitated, and the body absorbs more iron.

As can be seen from the data in Table 8.2, absorption of iron from iron salts, heme (blood) in meats, iron as ferritin in meat, or in a mixture of vegetables with meat-iron is increased (Moore, 1968). Diet and absorption interact to allow for greater absorption so long as the depletion is present. The criteria set for true nutritional adaptation have been met (Waterlow, 1985). Negative balance becomes positive balance without a change in iron intake. During the period of depletion, the child shows no functional ill effects and with a restoration of iron stores, the iron balance reverts to the prior steady state.

Absorption of iron from a pure vegetable source (e.g., wheat, rice, and corn), however, is not enhanced. Thus, the child with little or no meat intake does not adapt well to negative iron balance. Vegetarians can compensate by the consumption of iron-rich legumes eaten concomitantly with ascorbic acid rich fruits and vegetables. However, the poor family using excess amounts of so-called junk foods are at special risk for iron deficiency; these diets simply lack iron.

PREVENTION OF IRON DEFICIENCY

With respect to health policies, the research reviewed here consistently points to one conclusion: Prevention is likely to be more effective than therapeutic interventions. Nutritional supplementation and medical care may be sufficient for primary prevention of the nutritional deficiencies and developmental lags associated with disadvantaged environmental conditions. However, these interventions alone cannot completely reverse behavioral deficiencies once undernutrition has occurred. As noted, evidence shows that iron therapy does not completely correct the lower test scores of children who had iron deficiency anemia as infants, either in infancy or at early school age. Thus prevention, rather than treatment, holds greater promise for eliminating behavioral and developmental ill effects.

It is relatively easy to prevent iron deficiency anemia in infancy as evidenced by its dramatic decline in the United States. This was a result of increases in breast-feeding, the iron-fortified formula and cereal, and the Supplemental Feeding Program for Women, Infants and Children (WIC), which provides nutritional supplementation to mothers and children at risk for adverse social circumstances and medical problems (Vazquez-Seoane et al., 1985; Yip et al., 1987).

Much has happened in the past 20 years to improve the iron status of young children from poorer families in the U.S. Figure 8.1 shows the change in prevalence of anemia from 9% of children presenting to a clinic for the first time in 1973 to 5% in 1984 (Yip et al., 1987).

Why has this change occurred? Formerly accepted recommendations, such as the preparation of infant formulas from evaporated milk, have been abandoned. The encouragement of breast-feeding is now a strong concern in the health community, and formula and cereal for infants are now iron-fortified. But the population that is most at risk for iron deficiency requires more than simple supplementation of a formula available for purchase. Nutritional customs have a life of their own, and many mothers in poor communities obtain their nutritional advice from their own mothers and grandmothers. As Bradley notes in chapter 20, reaching families for the purpose of changing food habits requires the cooperation of that person in the family who makes critical decisions—the "pivotal" person. Furthermore, food supplement programs cannot be fully effective if they are not available for all poor families. Writing in 1987, Stockman reported that the WIC program reached "only 25 to 30% of eligible women and children [with eligibility at 185% of poverty level]. . . . Funding for the WIC program has been reasonably consistent but always under the threat of budgetary cuts and never as adequate as it should be."

An additional concern is the excess number of low-birth-weight infants born in disadvantaged circumstances. Infants weighing less than 2,500 g at birth have inadequate iron stores to support the "catch-up" growth that is desired. They are at high risk for becoming iron defi-

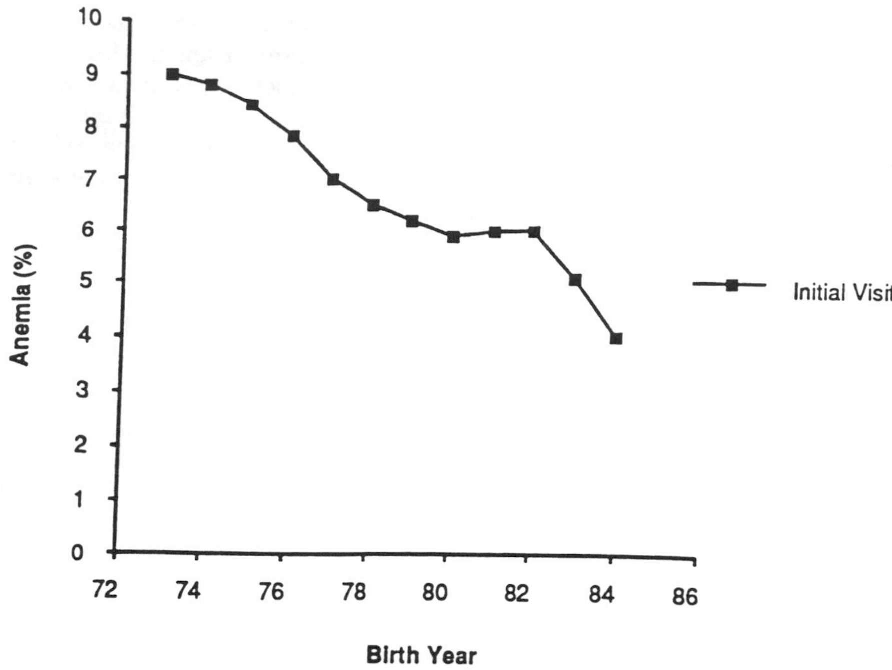

FIGURE 8.1 Prevalence of anemia (defined as Hgb < 10.3 g/dl for 6 months to 2 years of age and < 10.6 g/dl for 2 to 5 years of age) among children seen for the first time at the Pediatric Nutrition Surveillance Sites of the Centers for Disease Control.

From Yip et al. (1987).

cient with the deleterious effects described in this chapter. Providing 1 cc of multivitamin with iron to these children for the first 6 months of life, in addition to recommending breast-feeding or iron-fortified formula, will supply the additional 2 to 3 mg/kg of iron recommended.

The enhancement of absorption by ascorbic acid does influence iron absorption from legumes and grains. In Scandinavia, it is suggested that families reserve one meal for meats and legumes (both high in mineral content) with vegetables and fruits high in ascorbic acid content (Dallman, 1986). Dairy products are excluded from this one meal, thus preventing competition for absorption with other divalent cations such as calcium and zinc. Diets appropriate for the prevention of iron deficiency are presented in chapter 19.

Finally, the adaptive nature of iron metabolism in childhood gives the health care provider an opportunity to diagnose iron depletion and iron deficiency without anemia before there are observable consequences. Screening disadvantaged children for hemoglobin level and EP should be performed in the second 6 months of life and yearly thereafter. Further discussion of problems of identification of iron deficient children can be found in Herbert (1987) and in the report of the Expert Scientific Working Group (1985).

The finding of a child with iron deficiency anemia should alert the health care team that there are nutritional and, at times, social concerns to be addressed in the family (see Karp et al., 1974, 1984). Undernutrition is not an isolated occurrence in the life of a disadvantaged child. A full evaluation for iron deficiency, lead poisoning, and concomitant social and economic problems in the family should follow the determination of an elevation in EP in one child. The synergism among learning failure, poverty, and the environment that produces both poverty and learning failure should be considered. These issues are discussed extensively by Wachs, Sewell, Price, and Karp in other chapters in this text.

REFERENCES

Bayley, N. (1969). Bayley Scales of Infant Development Manual. New York: Psychological Corporation.

Crosby, W. H. (1976). Pica: A compulsion caused by iron deficiency. *Br Med J Haematology, 34*, 341–342.

Dallman, P. (1986). Iron deficiency in the weanling: A nutritional problem on the way to resolution. *Acta Pediat Scan, 323*(Suppl.), 59–67.

Expert Scientific Working Group. (1985). Summary of a report on assessment of the iron nutritional status of the United States population. *Am J Clin Nutrition, 42*, 1318–1330.

Herbert, V. (1987). Recommended daily intakes (RDI) of iron in humans. *Am J Clin Nutrition, 45*, 679–686.

Idjradinata, P., & Pollitt, E. (1993). Reversal of developmental delays in iron-deficient anaemic infants treated with iron. *Lancet, 341*, 1–4.

Judisch, J. M., Naiman, J. L., & Oski, F. A. (1966). The fallacy of the fat, iron deficient infant. *Pediatrics, 37*, 987–990.

Karp, R. J., Haaz, W. S., Starko, K., & Gorman, J. (1974). Iron deficiency in families of iron deficient inner-city school children. *Am. J. Dis. Child., 128*, 18–20.

Karp, R. J., Snyder, E., Fairorth, J. W., et al. (1984). Parental behavior and the availability of foods among undernourished inner-city children. *J Fam Practice, 18*, 731–735.

Lanzkowsy, P. (1959). Investigation into the aetiology and treatment of pica. *Arch Dis Child, 134*, 140–148.

Lozoff, B. (1989). Iron and learning potential in childhood. *Bullet. NY Acad Med, 65*, 1050–1066.

Lozoff, B. (1990). Has iron deficiency been shown to cause altered behavior in infants? In J. Dobbing (Ed.), *Brain, behavior, iron in the infant diet* (pp. 107–131). London: Springer Verlag.

Lozoff, B., & Brittenham, G. M. (1985). Behavioral aspects of iron deficiency. *Progr Hematol, 14*, 23–53.

Lozoff, B., Brittenham, G. M., Wolf, A. W., et al. (1987). Iron deficiency anemia and iron therapy effects on infant developmental test performance. *Pediatrics, 79*, 981–995.

Moore, C. V. (1968). Symposia of the Swedish Nutrition Foundation: VI. In G. Blix (Ed.), *Occurrence, causes and prevention of nutritional anemias* (p. 96). Stockholm: Amqvist & Wiksell.

Oski, F. (1979). The nonhematologic consequences of iron deficiency. *Am J Dis Child, 133*, 315–322.

Owen, G. M., Kram, K. M., Garry, P. J. et al. (1974). A study of the nutritional status of preschool children in the United States, 1968–1970. *Pediatrics, 53* (Suppl.), 597–646.

Stockman, J. A. (1987). Iron deficiency anemia: have we come far enough? *JAMA, 258*, 1645–1647.

Ten State Nutrition Survey. (1971). Ten State Nutrition Survey in the United States, 1968–1970: Preliminary Report to Congress. Atlanta: Public Health Service Centers for Disease Control.

Vazquez-Seoane, P., Windom, H., & Pearson, H. (1985). Disappearance of iron-deficiency in a high risk population given supplemental iron. *New Eng J Med, 313*, 1239–1240.

Walter, T., deAndraca, I., Chadud, P., et al. (1989). Adverse effect of iron deficiency anemia on infant psychomotor development. *Pediatrics, 84*, 7–17.

Waterlow, J. C. (1985). What do we mean by adaptation? In K. Blaxter, & J. C. Waterlow (Eds.), *Nutritional adaptation in man* (pp. 1–13). London: John Libbey.

Yip, R., Binken, N. J., Fleshhood, L., et al. (1987). Declining prevalence of anemia among low income children in the United States. *JAMA, 258*, 1619–1623.

9

Prevention and Treatment of Lead Poisoning

Paul Harris, MD, Margaret Clark, MD, and Robert J. Karp, MD

Lead poisoning in children is both theoretically and practically preventable. It is a disease that has received much attention from health providers and basic scientists alike, but little concerted action from the public or government. Although recently there has been a new emphasis on varied sources of lead in the environment including air, water, and dust, these elements contribute only a minute fraction to total lead absorption in children as compared with the major offender—lead-based paint. Lead-based paint still covers the walls of dilapidated prewar housing and serves as the major source of poisoning for poor children living in these substandard dwellings (Committee on Environmental Hazards, 1987; Environmental Defense Fund, 1990).

The clinical picture of lead poisoning has changed in the last three decades; it is rare now to see a child with overt encephalopathy. This change may reflect the impact of current standards for screening of and chelation therapy for children and for lead hazard abatement. We should not, however, be complacent about this more benign mask on the face of the lead hazard. We are now uncovering a veritable epidemic of low-level lead poisoning, which has subtle but permanent effects on learning and socialization skills. "Once success in those key [early school] years is gone," notes John Rosen (Hilts, 1990), "it's gone forever" (see chapter 3 and Rosen, 1985). This new epidemic demands new approaches with more emphasis on primary prevention.

MAGNITUDE OF THE EPIDEMIC

The National Health and Nutrition Examination Series II (NHANES II) of 1976 to 1980 estimated that at least 600,000 children 6 months to 5 years of age have blood lead (BPb) levels equal to or greater than 30 μg/dl (Mahaffey et al., 1982). Black children were dramatically overrepresented; 18% of black children living in the inner city had high Bpb levels as compared with 4% of children overall. This is harsh testimony to the effects of racial discrimination in housing. However, as with poverty in general, white children comprise about half the victims.

The Department of Health and Human Resources has recently extrapolated from the NHANES II data to estimate the number of children with lower levels of lead absorption that are now considered unacceptable (Mushak & Crosetti, 1989). At least 1.2 million children have BPb levels of 15 μg/dl or more, and each year, 400,000 fetuses are exposed to maternal BPb levels of 10 μg/dl or more.

WHAT HARM IS THERE IN A LITTLE LEAD?

Workers in the 1970s (Harris & Holley, 1972) demonstrated that lead crosses the placenta. More recently, Bellinger et al. (1987) showed sustained decrements in mental development in infants exposed to maternal BPb levels of 10 μg/dl or above. Needleman (1988), who has reviewed the breadth of research on lead and learning, draws the inescapable conclusion that even very low blood lead levels are associated with decreased cognitive and learning abilities, and motor skills (Deitrich, Berger & Succop, 1993). An example of this research is shown in Table 9.1.

Further, long-term follow-up studies of children treated for subclinical lead poisoning show repeated failures in school even among those children who received chelation therapy (Needleman & Gatsonis, 1990; Needleman et al., 1990). Current thinking is that there is no threshold for lead effects (Schwartz et al., 1990) and thus no "safe" BPb level. The *normal* BPb is zero.

CONSIDERATIONS OF LEAD AS AN ANTI-NUTRIENT

Human beings have not had sufficiently long experience with environmental lead to develop an adaptive response such as described for iron

TABLE 9.1 Lead Level in Deciduous Teeth (Parts per Million) and IQ Scores

Lead level	Mean Verbal IQ	
High >20	99.2	p value less than 0.05
Low <10	104.1	

From Needleman et al. 1985.

deficiency without anemia (see chapter 8). Lead, a toxic divalent cation, is treated by the body in ways that parallel the treatment of other minerals that serve as true nutrients. Moreover, in disadvantaged communities, lead is often available to children with a dietary deficiency of essential nutrients, especially iron.

There are three specific concerns. First, lead competes for absorption with other divalent cations such as calcium, iron, and zinc. Thus a dietary deficiency of one or all of these elements would enhance the absorption of lead and the likelihood of lead poisoning (Mahaffey, 1981). Moreover, as originally suggested by Lanzkowsky (1959), iron deficiency is often associated with pica, which, if lead is in the environment, will result in lead poisoning. Treatment of lead-poisoned children includes providing therapeutic doses of iron and encouraging a well-balanced diet that includes sufficient calcium, iron, and zinc. (Several chapters in part 3 address the need for social support to obtain nutritious food.)

Second, lead impairment of heme synthesis compounds the effect of iron deficiency, resulting in severer anemia and microcytosis than found with either disturbance alone (Clark et al., 1988). As shown in Table 9.2, there is also synergism between iron deficiency and lead poisoning in producing elevations in zinc-bound protoporphyrin (ZPP).

Third, lead poisoning and iron deficiency each contribute independently to learning failure among children. However, when these conditions coexist, children are 4 times more likely to show symptoms usually attributed to lead poisoning alone (Clark et al., 1988). The two curves shown in Figure 9.1 represent the distribution of IQs of groups of children with or without appreciable lead exposure. IQ in this example could represent any of a variety of measures of psychosocial or motor development. As shown by Needleman et al. (1990), low lead exposure with a serum lead between 25 and 40 pg/dl is associated with a 5-point drop in the mean IQ, accounting for numerous confounding social variables.

TABLE 9.2 Hemoglobin, Mean Corpuscular Volume (MCV) and Zinc Bound Protoporphyrin (ZPP) as Function of Iron Status Among Children With BPb >85 μg/dl

	Iron Status		
	Deficient	Marginal	Adequate
MCV (microliters)	56	61	74
Hemoglobin (g/dl)	8.9	10.1	11.4
ZPP (μg/dl)	693	581	240

All $p < 0.01$
From Clark et al, 1988. See chapter 8 for a full discussion of classifications of iron nutriture.

The exposure of children to lead has the potential to complicate nutritional guidance in other ways. For example, it is prudent to reduce the fat content of the diet to 30% of calories. A concomitant advantage would be the decreased absorption of lead (Mahaffey, 1981). By contrast, another prudent suggestion, to reduce intake of sodium ion, has a potentially harmful effect, as reduction in mineral ion intake (not just iron) increases the potential for pica to occur (see chapter 18).

An additional "dietary" source of lead requires mention—the containers in which food is stored or served. When families put acidic beverages (e.g., apple cider or orange juice) into crockery fired at low temperatures, there is a possibility of lead ion leaching from the glaze into the beverage. This inexpensive pottery, known as "software," is used unknowingly by poor, less educated families. The leaching of lead will not occur with the use of high-fired stoneware or porcelain. Moreover, for reasons of cost, convenience, or custom, poorer families are likely to have an increased risk of exposure from the consumption of canned fruits and vegetables as the lead content is considerably higher than that of fresh foods (Sills et al., 1991).

On a positive note, as suggested by the work of Clark et al. (1988), the declining occurrence of lead poisoning in the United States, even with persistent problems of lead in the environment, may reflect the availability of iron-fortified formulas as provided to infants by the Supplemental Food Program for WIC. Good body stores of iron are maintained, and, thus, lead absorption is inhibited.

SCREENING FOR LEAD POISONING

Our current practice is to screen children for evidence of undue lead absorption. Though more manageable than the screening of dwellings, this is sec-

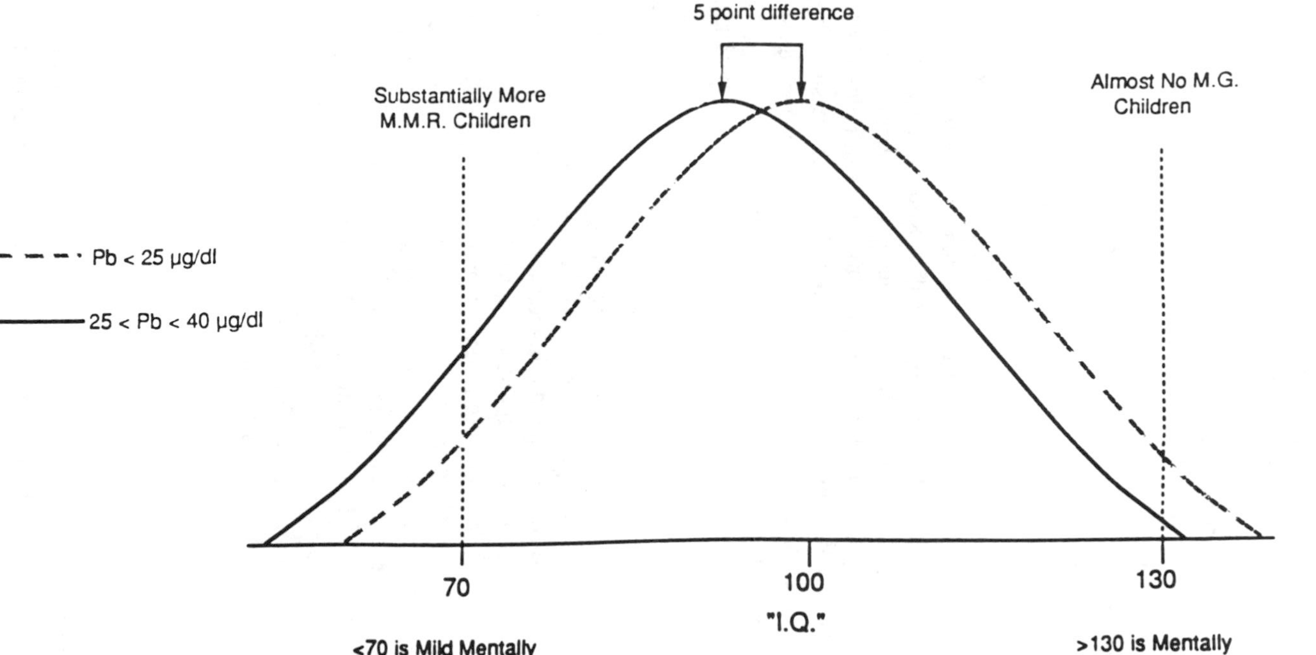

FIGURE 9.1 A downward shift in mean IQ score of 5 points may have little effect on the life of an individual child, but the effect on the community is essentially to empty the mentally gifted (M.G.) classes where children have an IQ two standard deviations above the mean (>130). The small change at the mean causes the classes for children who are mild mentally retarded (M.M.R.)—IQ two standard deviations below the mean(<70)—to become full to capacity.

ondary prevention at best. Because screening children will remain the practice for the foreseeable future, we suggest measuring BPb directly. Previously, a two-stage screening strategy, with initial ZPP measurements in the field, was suited for identifying children with BPb > 40 μg/dl; such a strategy will miss a substantial number of children with BPb in the 15- to 30-μg/dl range. In the past, the use of finger stick specimens collected on filter paper for measurement of BPb was rejected because surface contamination with lead was so common. This reservation may no longer apply because our current goal is to identify all children with exposure to lead. Lead on their fingers means lead is in their environment—which is what we are seeking to know.

Much more emphasis on screening and repairing housing before occupancy by children is required. An environmental history must be taken during routine health evaluations. It is important to know the age of the residence, the condition of the windows, the presence of structural damage, as well as the standard question: Is there any peeling paint and plaster? It is equally important to ask about places children frequent outside the home, such as day care or relatives' houses. In poorer communities, many baby sitters are unlicensed, and their homes are not inspected.

New York City has a new ordinance that mandates repairs of peeling paint for any pre–1960 building that is rented to families with children under 6 years of age—without regard to the lead status of the children. When people rue the possibility of "changing the system," they should remember that a coalition of health professionals and concerned laymen (The New York Coalition to End Lead Poisoning) was instrumental in getting inspection for lead paint included in the periodic inspection of city-owned dwellings. This is a model for efforts encouraged in chapter 26.

Although all preschool children living in pre–World War II–period housing should be screened for lead poisoning, two subgroups of children are at particularly high risk: (a) children whose parents are undocumented immigrants living in the most substandard housing, but who are afraid to seek help or medical care for fear of deportation; and (b) children of home owners with limited incomes who cannot afford to maintain their own property or, worse yet, are putting "sweat equity" into renovating a seriously dilapidated building while in residence (Clark et al., 1987).

MANAGEMENT OF ASYMPTOMATIC CHILD WITH LEAD POISONING

When a child is identified with an elevated BPb level, the essential task is to remove the child *immediately* and *permanently* from the source of lead.

The role of chelation therapy for children with moderately elevated BPb (between 15 and 40 μg/dl) is equivocal. There is no good evidence that the neurological sequelae of low lead exposure are reversible by chelation (Chisholm, 1987), and there is laboratory evidence that chelation may exacerbate the neurotoxicity by raising lead levels in neural tissue (Cory-Slecta et al., 1986). Children who continue to live in unsafe houses have persistently elevated BPb levels despite aggressive chelation (Chisholm, 1987). Moreover, there is also a tendency for parents and public health personnel alike to equate chelation with treatment. This attitude defers efforts to secure a safe environment for the exposed child. To give an example, the New York City Department of Health's (1985) *Guide for Childhood Lead Poisoning and Screening and Follow-up*, a 15-page document, devotes one footnote to environmental assessment.

The essential task of removing the child from the source of lead is easier to articulate than to accomplish. One primary concern is to be sure that the child is not in the dwelling during the process of deleading. The repair work creates lead dust, which increases the bioavailability of the lead (Sayres, 1987). Several alternatives to remaining in the home are available: hospitalizing the child, finding a relative with a lead-free home, setting up a municipal "safe house" for the entire family during the renovation period. Each of these options has difficulties attached, but one of them must be chosen, because the child cannot remain in the home during repairs.

A second concern is the lack of quality control in the deleading process. For instance, in New York City, the Department of Health accepts the landlord's repair work as adequate so long as it is done eventually. They do not stipulate that the workers be trained, that rooms be sealed, and carpets and bedding covered; or that the lead-bearing waste be disposed of properly. Nor are there safety standards for those who do the work.

A third concern is the lack of knowledge about the best way to delead a dwelling. There is recent evidence that the current practice of sanding or stripping lead-covered surfaces increases the lead content of house dust (Chisholm, 1986; Farfel & Chisholm, 1990; Sayre, 1987). Children returned to such homes have persistent elevations in BPb levels in the 30- to 40-μg/dl range. One important source of lead is in the window framing and sills that yield dust containing 200 times the accepted safety limit of lead. Deleading must include replacing windows and frames. More research is needed on the best ways to seal lead permanently rather than remove the lead containing paint in a manner that is analogous to the current approach to asbestos abatement (L. Cladzynski, 1986).

SUMMARY

Poverty and discrimination have created a high-risk environment for black children in the United States (United States Bureau of the Census, 1983, 1985). Lead poisoning is not a coincidental occurrence in their lives, but rather it is a product of a racial division of labor, unemployment, and underemployment in the job sector traditionally held by native-born African Americans. Moreover, institutional racism as expressed by discriminatory patterns for renting or selling housing (known as "redlining") has been the common practice in the urban United States. Traditionally, families have been denied mortgages when they attempt to purchase housing outside their assigned districts in black ghettos.

Lead poisoning is a family disease and a paradigm for the social, economic, and nutritional ills that befall the poor. They live in houses with old paint and on streets with traffic and lead containing air and dust. Because mouthing behavior is appropriate in infancy, *all* poor children living in or visiting old buildings are at risk for lead poisoning.

What then are the pragmatic and successful approaches to the prevention of lead poisoning? Prevention must go beyond the usual psychological, educational, and social support for children and families already affected to strategies that are largely political in nature. Such strategies may involve the health care community in unfamiliar activities: (a) supporting enactment and enforcement of strong antilead laws, (b) providing evidence for and serving as expert witnesses in individual and class-action suits seeking financial damages against slum landlords, and (c) giving public support to direct action of victims including rent strikes and public protests.

Lead, a known poison, should not be in the environment of any child. The environmental presence of lead, not occurring at all by chance, is of great consequence to children in our society, with African-American children bearing the greatest burden. What is called for is action to deal with the economic, social, and political problems that result in discrimination and poverty.

ACKNOWLEDGMENT

The authors thank Joseph Capella, MD, for his help in preparing this chapter.

REFERENCES

Bellinger, D., Levitan, A., Wateraux, C., & Needleman, H. (1987). Longitudinal analysis of prenatal and postnatal lead exposure and early cognitive development. *New England Journal of Medicine, 316*, 1037–1043.

Chisholm, J. J., Jr. (1986). Removal of lead paint from old housing: The need for a new approach. *American Journal of Public Health, 76*, 236–237.

Chisholm, J. J., Jr. (1987). Mobilization of lead by calcium disodium Edetate: A reappraisal. *American Journal of Diseases of Children, 141*, 1256–1257.

Cladzynski, L. (1986). Manual for the identification and abatement of environmental lead hazards (p. 19). Washington, DC: Health Resources and Services Administration, U.S. Public Health Service.

Clark, M., Harris, P., & Ajl, S. (1987). Failure to de-lead child's environment: A class analysis of children re-exposed to lead. Presented at the Annual Meeting of the American Public Health Association, New Orleans, LA.

Clark, M., Royal, J., & Seeler, R. (1988). Interaction of iron deficiency and lead and the hematologic findings in children with severe lead poisoning. *Pediatrics, 81*, 247–254.

Committee on Environmental Hazards/Committee on Accidents and Poison Prevention. American Academy of Pediatrics. (1987). Statement on lead poisoning. *Pediatrics, 79*, 457–465.

Cory-Slecta, D. A., Weiss, B., & Cox, C. (1987). Mobilization and redistribution of lead over the course of calcium disodium ethylene diamine tetra-acetate chelation therapy. *J Pharmacol Exeprimental Therapeutics, 243*, 804–813.

Deitrich, K. N., Berger, O. G., & Succop, P. A. (1993). Lead exposure and the motor developmental status of urban six-year-old children in the Cincinnati prospective study. *Pediatrics, 91*, 301–307.

Environmental Defense Fund. (1990). *Legacy of lead: America's continuing epidemic of childhood lead poisoning.* Washington, DC.

Farfel, M. R., & Chisholm, J. J., Jr. (1990). Health and environmental outcomes of traditional and modified practices for abatement of residential lead-based paint. *American Journal of Public Health, 80*, 1240–1245.

Harris, P., & Holley, M. R. (1972). Lead levels in cord blood. *Pediatrics, 49*, 606–608.

Hilts, P. J. (1990, December 20). U.S. opens a drive to wipe out lead poisoning among children. *New York Times*, p. 1.

Mahaffey, K. R. (1981). Nutritional factors in lead poisoning. *Nutrition Reviews, 39*, 353–360.

Mahaffey, K. R., Annest, J. L., Roberts, J., & Murphy, R. S. (1982). National estimates of blood lead levels: United States 1976–80. *New England Journal of Medicine, 307*, 373–379.

Mushak, P., & Crocetti, A. F. (1989). Determination of numbers of lead-exposed American children as a function of lead source: Integrated summary of a Report to the U.S. Congress on Childhood Lead Poisoning. *Environ. Res., 50*, 210–229.

Lanzkowsky P. (1959). Investigation into the aetiology and treatment of pica. *Archives of Diseases in Childhood, 34*, 140.

Needleman H. (1988, December). The persistent threat of lead: The medical and sociological issues. *Current Problems in Pediatrics*, 702–744.

Needleman, H. L., & Gatsonis, C. A. (1990). Low-level lead exposure and the IQ of children. *Journal of the American Medical Association, 263*, 673–678.

Needleman, H. L., Geiger, S. K., & Frank, R. (1985). Lead and IQ scores: A reanalyses. *Science, 227*, 701–704.

Needleman, H. L., Schell, A., Bellinger, D., et al. (1990). The long term effects of exposure to low doses of lead in childhood: An 11-year follow-up report. *New England Journal of Medicine, 322*, 83–88.

New York City Department of Health. (1985). *Guidelines for lead screening and follow-up.*

Rosen, J. F. (1985). Metabolic and cellular effects of lead: A guide to low level lead toxicity in children. In K. R. Mahaffey (Ed.), *Dietary and environmental lead: Human health effects* (pp. 157–185). New York: Elsevier.

Sayre, J. W. (1987). Deleading houses: Dangers in the dust. *American Journal of Diseases of Children, 141*, 727–728.

Schwartz, J., Landrigan, P. J., Baker, E. L., Jr., et al. (1990). Lead-induced anemia: Dose-relationships and evidence for a threshold. *American Journal of Public Health, 80*, 165–168.

Sills, M. R., Mahaffey, K. R., & Silbergeld, E. K. (1991). Lead levels in canned and fresh fruit. *New England Journal of Medicine, 324*(letter), 416–417.

United States Bureau of the Census. (1985). Characteristics of the population below the poverty level (1983) and Current Populations Reports (Series P-20). Washington, DC: U.S. Census Bureau, Government Printing Office.

10

Fetal Alcohol Syndrome

Robert J. Karp, MD,
Qutub Qazi, MD, PhD,
Joan Hittleman, PhD, and
Linda Chabrier, MD

When the dysmorphic features of children seem to have a common origin, the appearance is labeled a syndrome. What was formerly the most common grouping of children with dysmorphic features, Down syndrome, is a consequence of excessive genetic material from chromosome 21. Other syndromes are caused by teratogens including the specific toxic substance of concern in this chapter, alcohol (Brent & Beckman, 1990). Currently, Fetal Alcohol Syndrome (FAS) is the most common recognizable pattern of malformation.

But recognition of FAS is quite recent (Jones, Smith, Ulleland, et al., 1973). The disorder is a clinical diagnoses made when the characteristic dysmorphic features (see Figure 10.1), and developmental and physical delay are associated with a history of alcohol consumption in pregnancy (Streissguth, 1986). It is difficult to establish the overall incidence of FAS. Its individual features are quite common and "normal," because intrauterine exposure to alcohol is the usual occurrence in the United States. Although the dysmorphic features can occur on exposure to other toxic substances (Brent & Beckman, 1990), the consequences of FAS are detectable even in the absence of dysmorphic features (Kyllerman et al., 1985). This phenomenon is referred to as fetal alcohol effect (FAE).

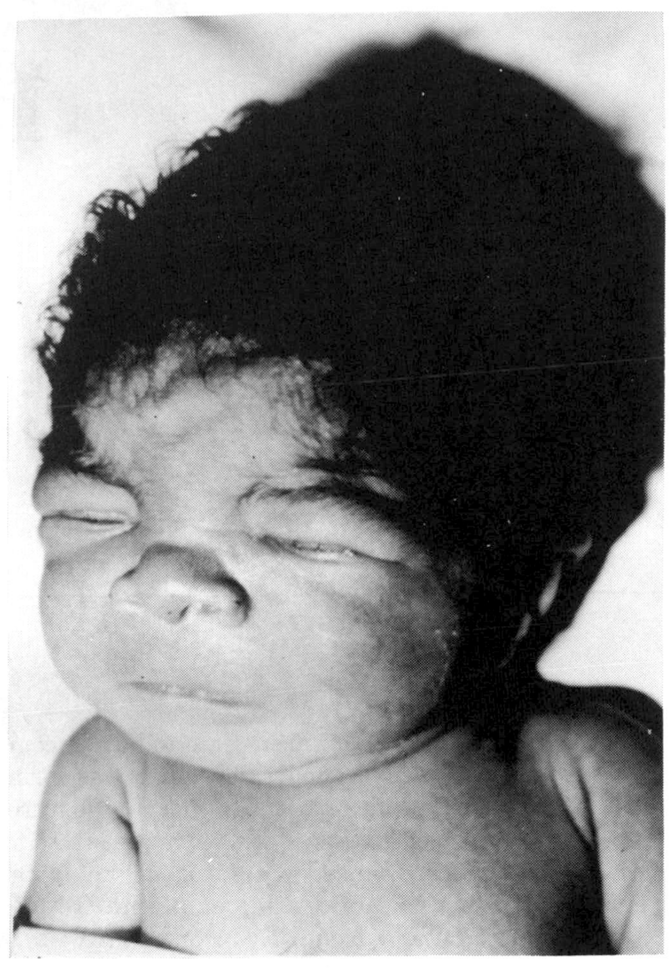

FIGURE 10.1 Characteristic facial dysmorphism in newborn infant with fetal alcohol syndrome.

The diagnosis of FAS requires the following (Clarren & Smith, 1978):
1. A history of maternal alcohol consumption during pregnancy.
2. Evidence of effects on somatic growth (e.g., a decrease in measures of height/length and/or weight for age and sex). Weight and head circumference are often disproportionately affected in FAS.
3. Evidence of effects on central nervous system (e.g., behavioral and/or intellectual development and/or decreased head circumference).
4. Features of the dysmorphology (e.g., absent philtrum, long upper lip, short palpebral fissures, etc.)

As noted in the introduction to this book, in utero exposure to alcohol contributes to transgenerational deprivation. FAS and FAE are associated with severe developmental consequences that interact with the social environment that produces FAS and FAE (alcoholism and poverty) to continue the cycle of poverty and deprivation (Karp, Qazi, Davis & Angelo, 1993). This is a "nature" *cross* "nurture" rather than "nature" *versus* "nurture" model.

FAS and FAE are not treatable diseases in the literal sense. This chapter presents the prevalence of alcohol use and abuse in the United States and addresses four ways that health care providers can help families address the problems of FAS children, for example, how to (a) make an early diagnosis, (b) identify the alcoholic mother, (c) counsel children living with alcoholic parents, and (d) advise women contemplating pregnancy. A comprehensive discussion of FAS and its consequences can be found in Streissguth (1986 and 1991).

THE PREVALENCE OF ALCOHOL USE AND ABUSE IN THE UNITED STATES

Social drinking is an accepted part of the lives of most Americans. Mean alcohol intake in the United States provides 5 to 7 percent of the nation's aggregate caloric needs (Lieber & Shaw, 1988). This is well within the capacity of the liver to metabolize alcohol. However, approximately one third of Americans do not drink at all (Russell, 1986). Another third drink at the acceptable level (less than 30 grams of ethanol per day), and roughly a third of all Americans drink excessively.

The control of social drinking requires a long period of cultural adaptation. Each alcohol-using culture has its own way of preventing drunkenness or social disability. Most cultures apply limits to drinking at various social occasions, whether the party is for cocktails or beer off the end of a pick-up truck. Even men who while their time away in neighborhood bars abide by a social code that limits their drinking. Alcohol consumption among Native Americans, however, presents another story.

Native Americans are a diverse group, yet they do share commonalities. The arrival of the Europeans first disrupted and then later destroyed the cultures established by these peoples. The disruption came with the introduction of horses, manufactured goods, fire-arms, and "fire-water"—alcohol. Some Native American tribes have gained control of the drinking problem. May et al. note ". . . . to a greater degree than with other adults in the United States, a great number of Indians quit drinking after age 30. Unfortunately, some of those who drink may become casualties before they quit or change from a flamboyant recreational style of consumption" (1988). Within Native American communities where control has been established, those ostracized from their social group by their relentless drinking reinforce their separation by excessive alcohol consumption. With women, continued drinking poses an additional threat, because the infants of older women suffer the greatest risk of developing FAS.

For Native Americans, the risk of FAS infants ranges from a low of 1.3 per 1,000 live births among the Navajo to 10.3 per 1,000 live births among Plains Indians (May et al., 1988). International data suggest that 1 in every 600 to 700 babies in the general population (1.3 per 1,000 live births) are born with the stigmata of FAS with an equal number of children showing effects of in utero exposure (Streissguth, 1986). The study by Marino et al. (1987) in the schools of an industrial town suggests that 10% of the children have some expression of alcohol exposure in utero.

WAYS THAT HEALTH CARE PROVIDERS CAN HELP FAMILIES ADDRESS THE PROBLEMS OF FAS CHILDREN

Early Diagnosis of FAS

The characteristic facial dysmorphism in a newborn infant are shown in Figure 10.1. It is unusual to find all the major features of the syndrome (Clarren & Smith, 1978; Hanson et al., 1976). The variability of phenotype may result from differences in dose of alcohol, age, and nutritional status of the mother (May, 1988), variations in timing of exposure, and genetic background of the fetus (Jones, 1991).

In a study conducted in Brooklyn, clinical data were collected on 92 children with FAS. The children were identified by their physical characteristics as well as a history of prenatal exposure to alcohol. Of 80 mothers, 34 were described as chronic alcoholics, 44 as heavy drinkers, 2 as moderate drinkers, and the remaining 7 refused to provide this information.

The typical mother of the FAS patient was an alcoholic or heavy drinker and older than 25 years of age. Moreover, she was of high parity, suffering from health problems secondary to alcoholism but lacking in adequate prenatal care, and often addicted to tobacco and other drugs of abuse. Prematurity and intrauterine growth retardation were

TABLE 10.1 CAGE Instrument

C—Have you ever had a need to Cut back on your drinking?
A—Have people Annoyed you because of your drinking?
G—Have you felt Guilty about your drinking?
E—Have you ever needed to start the day with a drink?
(an Eye opener)

Note: An alternative questionnaire substitutes "Tolerance" of alcohol (not feeling effects with the consumption of modest quantities) for "Guilt" in the CAGE.

commonplace prenatal occurrences. None of the infants were above the 50th percentile for birth weight, length, or head circumference and most were below the 10th percentile.

Sixty-four percent of the children presented with short palpebral fissures. Other important facial characteristics of these patients included hyertelorism; epicanthal folds; ptosis of the eyelids; strabismus; long philtrum with poor groove; micrognathia; a short nose with broad, flattened nasal bridge and anteverted nostrils; posteriorly rotated and/or low-set ears; and high-arched palate.

The finding of one or more of these fetal alcohol effects should be followed with careful investigation of the mother's drinking habits.

Identification of the Alcoholic Adult

Physicians have not been effective in identifying alcoholic parents even when the circumstances surrounding a child's life suggest social pathology (Duggan et al., 1991). Awareness and concern are essential (McDonald, 1991).

Bush and colleagues (1987) have shown that a well-conducted interview using the CAGE instrument has a high sensitivity, specificity, and positive predictive value in identifying the preclinical alcohol abuser—the person who consumes more than 60 grams of ethanol each day (four drinks). The question asked in administering the CAGE (see Table 10.1) is, "Do you drink at all?" However, the way one frames this question and administers the CAGE as a whole is crucial. The inquiry must be conducted in a relaxed manner without pen in hand so that a level of trust can be established between interviewer and interviewee. Ask yourself, "Will this information be used to provide help for the parent, or will this checklist be used in a court-mandated removal of a child from the home?" It would be inappropriate to use the CAGE in an adversarial situation, because this will destroy your relationship with the family.

CONSEQUENCE OF LIVING IN A HOME WITH AN ALCOHOLIC PARENT

The developmental disabilities of most children exposed in utero to alcohol must be considered in the context of the dysfunctions of the alcohol-abusing family. In essence, the child has four parents—drunk Mommy, sober Mommy, drunk Daddy, and sober Daddy. When Mom and Dad are sober, they may be wonderfully effective parents; however, the children in the family are never sure how long this state of affairs will last. These are children whose physical and emotional needs are met at random rather than with any consistency (Brown, 1986).

The greatest dilemma encountered by children of alcoholic parents is that they often feel personally responsible for their parent's habit, and this guilt becomes very difficult for them to handle. In addition, there is the burden and constant embarrassment when the child's young friends see the alcoholic parents, especially given how cruel and unforgiving young children can be. Some suggestions for children of alcoholic homes appear in a book entitled *I Know the World's Worst Secret* (Sanford, 1987). Children need to know that they are not to blame, can express emotions and reach out to other people, can protect themselves from physical danger caused by the drinking, and, above all, they can seek help for themselves and the family.

SOME ADVICE FOR THE MOTHER

What should a health care provider advise women about to become pregnant?

- FAS is a preventable but untreatable disease whose occurrence depends, in part, on inherited characteristics that cannot be predicted.
- The growth and neurological disabilities associated with alcohol consumption in pregnancy (both FAS and FAE) persist even when the child grows up in a good home. (See *The Broken Cord*, an account by Michael Dorris of his experience raising a son with FAS.)
- Poverty alone does not predict alcoholism, but poor women are at high risk for undernutrition, which increases vulnerabilty of the fetus to the effects of alcohol. These effects (FAE) provide additional impediments to learning in situations in which resources for recognition and rehabilitation are limited (see chapter 3).
- The provider should keep in mind that past drinking and dietary behavior may be kept hidden.

Thus, our recommendation, like Jones (1991), "is to counsel all women contemplating pregnancy to abstain from alcohol."

SUMMARY

It is intriguing to consider why the in utero effects of alcohol went unrecognized for so long. Smith (1977) and subsequently Streissguth (1986 & 1991) provide detailed histories of incomplete observations; the association of alcohol exposure and physical and developmental consequences were recognized, but the results were not followed with sufficient vigor to achieve general acceptance of causation—alcohol in pregnancy leads to FAS/FAE.

In the introduction to the text, we show that in the United States a compelling, though incorrect, explanation for "feeble-mindedness" in children of alcoholic parents was actively promoted. Mental retardation, it was said, caused alcoholism. The acceptance of this counter-hypothesis may provide partial explanation for the subsequent absence of curiosity about in utero alcohol effects (Karp, Qazi, Davis, & Angelo, 1993).

Children with FAS or FAE can be helped in their social adjustment by placement in good foster care or by having a birth mother who goes through rehabilitation and no longer drinks. It is essential to get help for these families because the children are vulnerable to the social pathology of the alcoholic family.

REFERENCES

Brent, R. L., & Beckman, D. A. (1990). Environmental teratogens. *Bulletin of NY Academy of Medicine, 66*, 123–163.

Brown, S. (1986). Children with an alcoholic parent. In N. J. Estes & M. E. Heinemann (Eds.), *Alcoholism: Development, consequences, and interpretations* (1st ed.) (pp. 207–220). St. Louis: Mosby.

Bush, B., Shaw, S., Cleary, P., et al. (1987). Screening for alcohol abuse using the CAGE questionnaire. *Am J Med, 82*, 231–235.

Clarren, S. K., & Smith, D. W. (1978). Fetal alcohol syndrome. *N Engl J Med, 298*, 1063–1067.

Dorris, M. (1989). *The broken cord.* New York: Harper & Row.

Duggan, A. K., Adger, H., Jr., McDonald, E. M., et al. (1991). Detection of alcoholism in hospitalized children and their families. *Am J Dis Child, 145*, 1317.

Hanson, J. W., Jones, K. L., & Smith, D. W. (1976). Fetal alcohol syndrome: Experience with 41 patients. *JAMA, 235*, 1458–1460.

Jones, K. L. (1991). Fetal alcohol syndrome. *Pediatrics in Review, 12*, 380–381.

Jones, K. L., Smith, D. W., Ulleland, C., et al. (1973). Patterns of malformation in offspring of chronic alcoholic mothers. *Lancet, i,* 1267.

Karp, R. J., Qazi, Q. H., Davis, J. M., & Angelo, W. A. (1993). Fetal alcohol syndrome at the turn of the 20th century: "hereditary feeble-mindedness" revisited. (Abstract) Meetings of the American Pediatric Society/Society for Pediatric Research. Washington, DC, May 3–6.

Kyllerman, M., Aronson, M., Sabel, K. G., et al. (1985). Children of alcoholic mothers: Growth and motor performance compared to matched controls. *Acta Pediat Scand, 74,* 20–26.

May, P. A., Hymbaugh, K. J., Aase, J. M., et al. (1988). Epidemiology of fetal alcohol syndrome among American Indians of the Southwest. *Social Biology, 30,* 374–385.

McDonald, D. I. (1991). Parental alcoholism: A neglected pediatric responsibility. *Am J Dis Child, 145,* 609–610.

Sanford, D. (1987). *I know the world's worst secret.* Oregon: Multinomah Press.

Smith, D. W. (1977). Fetal alcohol syndrome: A tragic and preventable disorder. In N. J. Estes & M. E. Heinemann (Eds.), *Alcoholism: Development, consequences, and interpretations* (1st ed.) (pp. 144–149). St. Louis: Mosby.

Streissguth, A. P. (1986). Fetal alcohol syndrome: An overview and implications for patient management. In Estes & Heinemann (Eds.), *Alcoholism: Development, consequences, and interpretations* (pp. 195–206). St. Louis: Mosby.

Streissguth, A. P., et al. (1991). Fetal alcohol syndrome in adolescents and adults. *JAMA, 265,* 1961.

11

Malnutrition in Children with Human Immunodeficiency Virus Infection

Hermann Mendez, MD, and
Simon Rabinowitz, MD, PhD

In the United States, the incidence of Acquired Immunodeficiency Syndrome (AIDS) in infants and children is increasing at an alarming rate. Most of the reported cases have occurred in the offspring of high-risk disadvantaged parents: intravenous (IV) drug abusers, prostitutes, and illegal immigrants from the Caribbean. Therefore, a growing cohort of the sickest pediatric patients in many urban hospitals is being discharged to parents who are financially, and often physically and emotionally, least able to deal with the demands of child rearing. One of the biggest problems they face is preventing the failure to thrive that plagues many of these infants and children.

This chapter begins with comments on the epidemiology, transmission, and clinical presentation of AIDS in children. The major focus of the chapter, however, is on the various factors that result in the wasting syndrome, frequently seen in pediatric AIDS. We then discuss the relationship between immunity and nutrition, and offer some dietary guidelines based on the literature and experience of the authors.

EPIDEMIOLOGY

As of April 1990, 2,192 cases of AIDS in children less than 13 years of age had been reported to the Centers for Disease Control, accounting for 1.7% of the total in the United States (Centers for Disease Controls, 1990). A large proportion (82%) of cases were associated with perinatal transmission. Since only AIDS cases are accounted for, this figure underestimates the true incidence of human immunodeficiency virus (HIV) infection in the pediatric population. Most of the pediatric cases are reported from cities on the East Coast, with New York reporting more than one quarter of the total, followed by New Jersey, Florida, California, and Puerto Rico.

In the United States 82% of pediatric AIDS cases were via vertical (perinatal) transmission, and 15% were via blood or blood products. Of perinatally acquired cases 51% were born to IV drug–using mothers; 21% to sexual partners of IV drug–using men; 18% to sexual partners of persons with HIV infection; 2% to mothers who had received transfusion, and in 8% of the mothers the route of HIV infection was undetermined. Unfortunately, overall mortality is exceedingly high with most of the deaths occurring during the first 2 years of life.

ROUTES OF TRANSMISSION

The probability of an infant born to an HIV seropositive mother being infected appears to be in the range of 20% to 35% (Goddert et al., 1989). Infants and children that require the transfusion of blood or blood products are at increased risk of transfusion-acquired HIV infection, but the highest exposure to HIV through transfusions occurred before 1986. Current blood donation practices and screening for HIV have significantly decreased the risk for transmission of the virus. In the future, new pediatric infections are unlikely to occur in this way. Mother-to-infant transmission will provide the overwhelming majority of new cases.

Of note, there are reports that breast-feeding can transmit HIV infection. The U.S. Public Health Service recommends that HIV-infected women avoid breast-feeding, but the World Health Organization does not recommend cessation of breast-feeding in developing countries, because it is the sole reliable source of nutrition in those countries. Children can acquire HIV infection as a result of sexual abuse, but most of the reports are anecdotal. The quantification of the frequency of transmission via this mechanism is obscured by the fact that HIV infection is oftentimes present in the mother as well.

BASIS FOR MALNUTRITION IN HIV INFECTION

There are three main causes for children to fail to thrive. The first, and most important in nearly all cases, is inadequate intake of nutrients. HIV-infected children are frequently sick with intercurrent illnesses. Regardless of the organ system primarily involved, a child who doesn't feel well will have a poor appetite and a poor intake of calories. The second factor is ineffective use of the calories ingested. Because there is a high prevalence of enteric infections in this patient population, malabsorption is frequently encountered. The malabsorption of an already compromised caloric intake yields inadequate energy and nutrients available to the growing child. Finally, these children who are receiving suboptimal calories for their age, weight, and size often have higher caloric requirements because of fever, tissue damage, and the other consequences of their infections. In summary, children with HIV infection often require more calories than their peers, but take in substantially less and use them less efficiently.

The major contributor to the malnutrition that results from HIV infection is the presence of enteric infection, which decreases oral intake and causes malabsorption. Children with AIDs are particularly susceptible to these infections because of a variety of problems in their immunological and gastrointestinal functions. The responsible organisms are both microbes found in the general population and opportunistic agents limited to immunocompromised hosts. To make matters worse, there is no effective antimicrobial therapy for some of the opportunistic infections frequently seen in the gastrointestinal tract. Infections with many of these organisms often result in villous atrophy, decreased intestinal absorptive capacity, and malabsorption syndromes.

Although infections in the gastrointestinal tract are not necessarily seen as "terminal" events, the child with a severely compromised ability to be alimented has a very grave prognosis. There is also an AIDS-associated enteropathy that is found in the absence of any identifiable organisms. This condition also decreases intake of nutrients and increases metabolic energy requirements. In adult patients it is related to lower anthropometric measurements, d-xylose malabsorption, steatorrhea, and histological abnormalities of the small intestine and colon. Regardless of the etiology, any substantial inflammatory process of the gastrointestinal tract will yield malabsorption. Therefore, children with HIV disease will often have diarrhea and generally have to take in additional calories to assimilate adequate quantities to grow.

Infections of the oropharynx and esophagus may cause substantial mouth pain and quickly lead to anorexia in children who are already weak and ill. Aside from enteric infections, other generalized infectious and noninfectious processes may also lead to anorexia. One common presenting manifestation of pediatric AIDs is recurrent, serious bacterial infections (sepsis, meningitis, arthritis, osteomyelitis, pneumonia, and organ abscesses). Encephalopathy in HIV infection may present as developmental delays, deterioration of motor skills, and behavioral abnormalities that compromise eating. Respiratory illnesses, common in children with HIV infection, also compromise appetite. The progressive hypoxia and tachypnea seen in these patients not only interfere with intake but also yield a higher basal metabolic rate, thus increasing caloric needs. In addition, other problems encountered in children with HIV disease can affect well-being and appetite. These include hepatitis, renal disease, and cardiomyopathy that can present as congestive heart failure.

NUTRITION AND IMMUNITY

Malnutrition itself has been associated with immune dysfunction in otherwise immunocompetent individuals. In developing countries where environmental factors lead to protein-calorie malnutrition there is an increased susceptibility to infection and disease, and nearly all of the body's defense mechanisms are impaired. Single nutrient deficiencies of zinc and selenium also impair immune function and have been shown to be reduced in adult patients with AIDS.

There are striking parallels between the ways in which the immune system is impaired in malnutrition and in HIV infection. It has been hypothesized that malnutrition is not just a sequelae of advanced AIDS enteropathy, but rather an early finding in HIV infection that plays a crucial role in the development of overwhelming opportunistic infection.

DIETARY SUGGESTIONS

The adult and pediatric literature generally convey a pessimistic prognosis toward alimenting patients with advanced AIDS, especially in the face of gastrointestinal tract disease. However, there have not been any investigations on the feasibility of preventing malnutrition, and any beneficial impact this might have on the course of the disease process.

Presently, the guidelines for alimenting children with AIDS are minimal (Falloon et al., 1989). Suggestions include intravenous alimentation when necessary and restriction of lactose in the diet because lactase deficiency is commonly found in the setting of intestinal disease.

The approach that we use in children with failure to thrive and pediatric AIDs is as follows: Initially a height, weight, and diet history with calorie counts is obtained. If diarrhea is present, stools are sent for investigation of infectious agents including fresh specimens for cryptosporidium. If there is no worsening of abdominal pain or diarrhea with dairy products or fatty foods, no restrictions are placed on the diet. Caloric intake is nearly always inadequate, and a nutritionist discusses with the primary caretaker food likes and dislikes of the child, and suggestions are offered to increase caloric intake. Regular follow-up (monthly or biweekly) is instituted.

Children who present with intractable diarrhea secondary to cryptosporidium or mycobacterium avian intracellulare present a difficult problem because effective antimicrobial therapy is not available. Clinical attempts to decrease gastrointestinal motility and secretion have been initiated.

If diarrhea and weight loss persist and all of the investigations for infectious agents are negative, then dietary restrictions are instituted. Stools are checked for reducing substances, pH, and fat to evaluate the type of malabsorption. If reducing substances are found, a test for lactose intolerance is performed. If it is positive, then dairy products are removed and either Lactaid® milk or drops, or lactose-free infant formula are started.

When weight loss in the absence of diarrhea is documented and all attempts to increase oral caloric intake have been unsuccessful, nasogastric tube feedings are used. The choice of formula is based on the oral intake and malabsorption pattern of the patient. In many situations a standard formula is used. All children are encouraged to eat. Once their appetite returns and oral intake increases, they are weaned from the supplemental feedings. For children who require nasogastric feedings, a concerted effort is made with the nursing staff and social workers to teach the technique to the caretaker or to provide home attendants so that the children may return home as soon as possible.

Certain children with advanced infectious or noninfectious enteropathy are unable to tolerate disaccharides, whole proteins, and long-chain triglycerides. They are placed on an "elemental" diet (e.g., constructed from amino acids and monosaccarides). Although some children will take small amounts of these products (after artificial flavoring has been added) orally, all children requiring these diets wind up with nasogastric tube feedings. We have found a few children who initially could not tolerate lactose, or who required elemental diets that improved with time and could begin more standard formulas. As mentioned, we have also had several children whose appetite improved after a period of tube feeding and were able to go back to an oral diet.

In our experience, nutritional intervention is most rewarding when it is initiated at the first signs of a problem. Children who are allowed to become too cachectic before the introduction of adequate nutrition uniformly do poorly. Certain centers use total parenteral nutrition in many of their patients with HIV disease. We reserve this therapy for the small number of children who are acutely too ill to tolerate enteral nutrition. In almost all cases this is viewed as a temporary therapy to be replaced by nasogastric feeding of elemental diets. In our experience, the risk of serious infection via the central line in these immunocompromised children is too great to be considered a permanent therapy.

REFERENCES

Centers for Disease Control. (1990, April). HIV/AIDS surveillance.

Falloon, J., Eddy, J., Wiener, L., & Pizzo, P. A. (1989). Human immunodeficiency virus in children. *Journal of Pediatrics, 114*, 1–9.

Goddert, J. J., Mendez, H., Drummon, J. E., et al. (1989). Mother to infant transmission of human immunodeficiency virus type 1: Association with prematurity or low anti-gp 120. *Lancet, 2*, 1015.

12

Obesity in Disadvantaged Children

M. R. C. Greenwood, PhD,
Patricia R. Johnson, PhD,
Robert J. Karp, MD, and
Patricia Giblin Wolman, EdD, RD
with contributions by
Joanne Hurley, MS, RD,
Edith Snyder, MS

Obesity has been identified as one of the largest public health and nutrition concerns in the United States since the 1970s (Bray, 1976). The Diet and Health Report of the National Research Council (1989) establishes that 31% of men and 25% of women older than 18 years of age in the United States are overweight. The Surgeon General's Report on Nutrition and Health (1988) included the statement that "Obesity is one of the most prevalent diet-related problems in the United States. It affects about 34 million adults." Additional estimates suggest that as many as 15% to 20% of school-age children are also overweight. Thus, it is the rare individual in our society who does not have an obese relative, friend, or acquaintance.

Although we commonly speak about obesity, investigators in the field are in general agreement that obesity is not a single, unitary disorder, but rather a collection of disorders that share the common feature of excess accumulation of fat tissue and a series of associated metabolic disorders (Callaway & Greenwood, 1984). There is also general consensus among health professionals that obesity carries with it increased health risks, measured both as increased morbidity and mortality, and as increased risk for specific disease states including cardiovascular disease, hypertension, non–insulin-dependent diabetes, certain forms of cancer, gallbladder disease, menstrual abnormalities, and complications of arthritis and gout (Rim & White, 1979). Furthermore, the distribution of body fat, as well as fatness per se, may contribute to risk for some disease states (e.g., cardiovascular disease). For example, it has been shown in a large population of women that incidences of myocardial infarction, stroke, and overall death are correlated with high waist to hip ratios, which reflect an upper-body, or abdominal, distribution of fat, as opposed to a lower-body, or femoral, distribution (Lapidus et al., 1986). Among the women who fell into the highest 20% for waist-to-hip ratio, the relative risk for myocardial infarction was 8.2 times greater than for women in the lowest 20% for waist-to-hip ratio. The epidemiological data on the relationships between body weight and risk for these chronic diseases in general follows a U- or J-shaped curve. In other words, mortality increases as body weight increases or decreases above the mean (National Research Council, 1989).

Because we understand obesity to be a complex multiple set of disorders, it is not surprising that we also find multiple factors that contribute to its etiology. These include nutritional, metabolical, endocrinological, and genetic factors, all of which are believed to be, in varying degrees, important contributors to the development of obesity.

Furthermore, the data derived from epidemiological studies lead to the conclusion that the prevalence of human obesity is strongly influenced by cultural and social determinants as well. Economic, racial, gender, and ethnic factors and their interactions produce diverse correlations with the prevalence of obesity in populations (Garn, 1986). For example, prevalence of obesity is exceptionally high in middle-aged women of low socioeconomic status, and in some particular racial and ethnic groups. Furthermore, American women who are black are at greater risk for becoming obese than their white counterparts matched for age and socioeconomic status (Van Itallie, 1985).

Although data gathered on experimental animals suggest that dietary fat, independent of total caloric intake, is a contributor to the development of obesity, there are no data that establish this effect in human populations (National Research Council, 1989). A few short-term studies suggest that a reduction of fat content in the diet may be accompanied by loss of body weight, but often in these reports, reduced caloric intake has occurred as well. Thus, it is possible that reducing total fat in the diet may lead to reduced caloric intake, perhaps because of differences in diet palatability. Furthermore, because both obesity and high-fat diets are independently correlated with increased risk for chronic disease, reduction in dietary fat is a rationale recommendation for populations at risk for obesity (National Research Council, 1989).

Another well-known observation about human obesity is that it tends to run in families, as well as in particular ethnic and social groups. Thus, obesity has long been considered to have a genetic component. It has been difficult, however, to tease apart the relative contributions of genetics and environment to the pathogenesis of obesity. Both twin and adoption studies have now established that genetic background has a major influence on the occurrence of obesity (Bouchard et al., 1981; Sorensen et al., 1988; Stunkard et al., 1986). The risk of becoming obese that is associated with parental obesity is more important than the family environment during childhood (Price et al., 1987). The recent elegant analyses of the various contributions of genetic and environmental factors on the risk of becoming obese carried out by Claude Bouchard (1989) clearly demonstrate that not only is genetic background itself important in the etiology of obesity, but also that genetic cross environmental interactions contribute significantly. These data strongly suggest that the sensitivity of individuals to increases in the amount of body fat following overfeeding are dependent on the individual's genotype.

These findings that establish a contribution for genetic background and genetic–environmental interactions should not discourage us from seeking effective strategies for both treatment and prevention of obesity. Rather, this knowledge should encourage a search for better means of treatment and prevention, because it will enable us to identify more easily particular populations of individuals that are at risk for obesity.

One such population that is at risk for obesity involves members of groups that are moving away from a status of deprivation. Semistarvation has been a common human experience shaping people's biologic (genetic) and environmental responses to both deprivation and plenty (Dietz & Gordon, 1981). People who have experienced starvation may overeat without awareness of the consequences of excess. Abundant data from studies of immigrant groups (Dietz & Gordon, 1981; Goldblatt et al., 1965), Native Americans (Knowler et al., 1981), and black and white Americans of various socioeconomic status (Van Itallie, 1985) suggest that obesity follows leanness when people rise from deprivation plus poverty to poverty alone.

Both wasting (decreased weight for height) and obesity are more common among children from the poorest and least educated families (Hamm et al., 1989). The most disadvantaged boys and girls, however, are on the average lean, but the girls tend to become obese when they reach adulthood (Gortmaker et al., 1987). Stanley Garn (1986) makes the following observation: "Among American adults, the relationship between socioeconomic status and fatness is curvilinear in both sexes, being the lowest below the poverty level, then rising to the poverty level among women and to middle income level in men, then falling again" (see Figure 12.1).

Among both men and women from the highest level of socioeconomic status, leanness is the rule. These observations suggest that obesity may be the first step away from deprivation. An important limitation of these observations, however, is that socioeconomic status itself, tells us little about the lives of individual families and children within any particular socioeconomic status group (Wachs & Gruen, 1982; see Wachs's comments in chapter 2). Poor communities are heterogeneous with respect to degree of deprivation and family life-style. It is necessary to show that children who show evidence of wasting live in situations of deprivation plus poverty, whereas poverty alone is associated with a full range of weight versus height ratios including those that suggest overweight and obesity.

Two data sets from impoverished inner-city communities contain such information: (a) When measured on entry into school, inner-city children whose parents delayed their children's entry into school were significantly leaner than children who entered school at an appropriate age (Karp et al, 1976). (b) Among preschool children, those who were abused were significantly leaner than their nonabused controls (Karp et al., 1989). In both of these studies, some of the children who came from the poverty-only situation were obese.

CASE STUDIES

The four case studies that follow illustrate some of the behaviors in poor families in which the caregiver appears to believe that overfeeding is the proper feeding for children. Examination of these cases can lead us to some generalizations about poverty life-style situations that may suggest common approaches for providing preventive guidance to lessen the probability of the development of obesity.

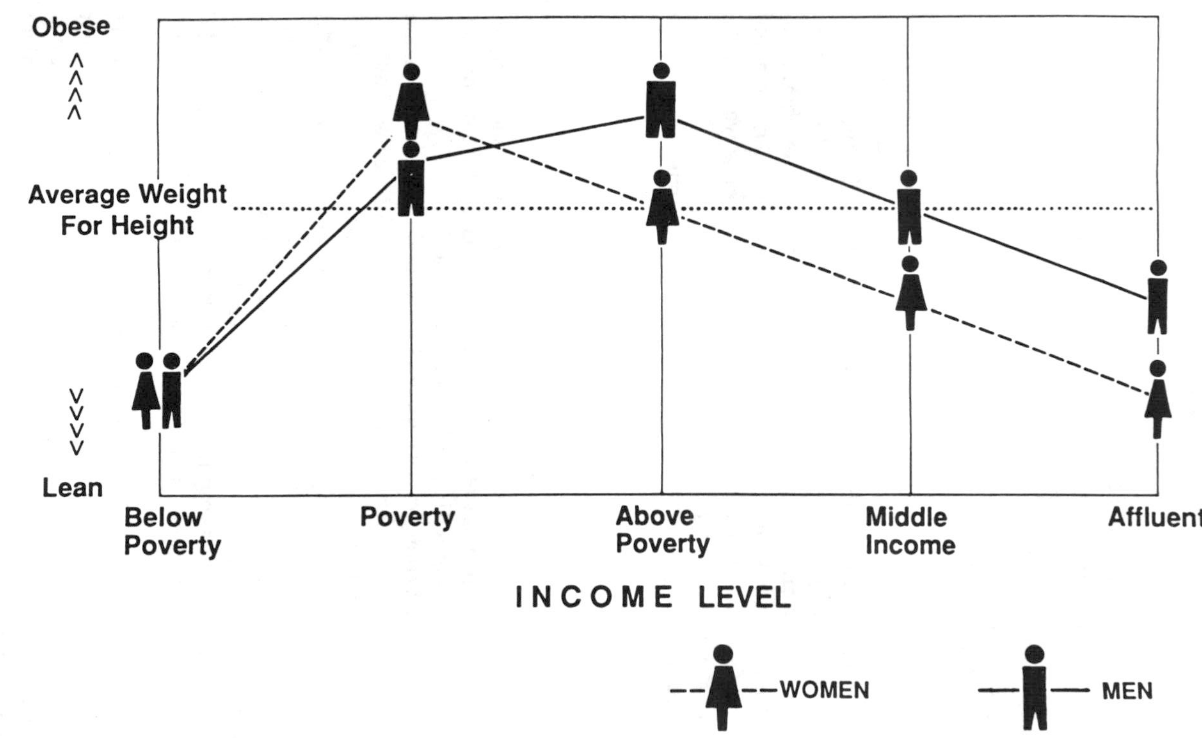

FIGURE 12.1 Relationship between socioeconomic status and obesity.

Adapted from Garn (1986).

Joel (from a New England family, both white and poor)

Patricia Gilman Wolman, EdD, RD

Sheila, Joel's mother, was the youngest of eight children. Her father, Vance, was a lobsterman who fished the Maine coast. He left lobstering after he had an experience with hypothermia resulting from a fall overboard from his boat. His boots filled with freezing water, and he was pulled under before being rescued. While he was being treated for this episode of hypothermia, he and his wife, Effie, decided to move to northern Maine where Effie had family, and they hoped that Vance could get a job with a lumber company. However, his developing arthritis made it impossible for him to work effectively in the cold climate. He had no pension or disability benefits, and settled for taking only odd jobs. Effie secured a job as a waitress in a fishing lodge in spring and summer. In the fall, she earned some money by making and selling Christmas wreaths. Because Sheila was the only one of their eight children still at home, they managed to put plenty of food on the table by maintaining a large garden and canning and freezing their abundant garden produce. Vance was able to supplement the family's diet by hunting and fishing.

Sheila hated their life in the woods. She missed her friends from the coast. Her parents were hurt and confused when she became pregnant during her junior year in high school. When Joel was born, Vance and Effie insisted that Sheila finish her schooling, and thus they became Joel's primary caretakers. Sheila became jealous of her parents' close relationship with Joel. Her son ignored her when his grandparents were there, and preferentially sought them out when he was hurt or needed help of any kind. Sheila dropped out of high school. She took Joel from her parents' home and moved in with another single mother.

Sheila got two part-time jobs to support herself and her son, and took a course that would enable her to get a high school equivalency diploma. Because of her income level she was entitled to food stamps but used them only once, finding the experience humiliating in a small town with only one place to shop for groceries. Sheila placed Joel in a Head Start program. Effie and Vance cared for Joel when Sheila worked odd shifts. Joel and his grandmother spent long winter afternoons and evenings watching television and baking in Effie's cozy kitchen. Joel loved to take home to his mother the cookies, muffins, pies, and cakes that he and his grandmother made.

Dr. Wolman first met Sheila when she enrolled in an Expanded Food and Nutrition Education Program (EFNEP). EFNEP is federally funded, but locally administered by land-grant universities in each state. Aides in the program are paraprofessionals who are taught to evaluate diets and to teach homemakers with young families meal planning, food purchasing, and food sanitation practices. EFNEP aides make individual home visits and teach homemakers in small groups, usually at the home of one of the participants in the program.

Several 24-hour-diet recalls taken by the EFNEP aide indicated that for breakfast Joel usually ate the cookies, muffins, or cakes that he had taken home from his grandmother's. He had lunch at Head Start and generally ate a hot dog on a roll or a bologna sandwich on white bread for dinner. He also snacked on sweets in the evening. On the average of twice each week, Sheila took Joel to the shopping mall where he had a cheeseburger, french fries, and ice cream at a fast-food restaurant. When Joel had dinner with his grandparents, the usual menu consisted of a creamy fish chowder, fried fish or meat (usually game), fried potatoes, a creamed vegetable, and cookies or cake for dessert. With the exception of his lunch at Head Start, Joel ate no fruits except blueberries or apples in pies or muffins. He ate vegetables only when he dined with his grandparents and had milk an average of three times per week.

Joel, who was not quite 4 years old, weighed 45 lb and was 40 in. in height, which placed him in the 90th percentile for weight and the 50th percentile for height.

The EFNEP aid helped Sheila plan more varied and nutritious meals. With Sheila's permission, the aide took an inventory of the food in the house and helped Sheila write a grocery list. Sheila's typical shopping pattern was to run into the store on her way home from work before she picked up Joel and buy whatever seemed appealing to her. Sheila had never seen her mother write a shopping list and thus it did not occur to her that she might use one. Joel loved sweets, so she bought him Kool-Aid® to drink. She never insisted that he drink milk or eat vegetables, and she tried to outdo her mother by buying the richest, creamiest baked goods that the "Stop and Shop" had to offer. She rarely kept milk in the house, because she did not drink it, and Joel did not drink it often enough. It usually soured and had to be thrown away. Sheila grew up in a household where all of the vegetables came from the garden; she rarely traveled down the aisles of the store where canned or frozen vegetables were displayed. Occasionally her mother gave her fresh vegetables. Although Sheila worried about Joel getting enough to eat, her lunch at work plus cookies or cake with coffee in the evening satisfied her appetite. She prepared hot dogs or bologna sandwiches for Joel because she thought that he should have some meat, he liked them, and they were easy to fix and did not spoil quickly.

The EFNEP aide suggested that Sheila buy some cold cereal and dried skim milk powder for Joel's breakfast. Sheila made her first grocery list. After the next home visit the aide reported that Joel liked having cereal for breakfast, but did not like the reconstituted skim milk. Sheila agreed to buy 2% fat milk in quarts, so it would be less likely to spoil. The aide encouraged Sheila to give Joel milk instead of Kool-Aid.® She also asked Sheila to save her grocery tapes so that they could compare the grocery lists they wrote together with what Sheila actually purchased. It was apparent that Sheila continued to buy treats impulsively, but she gradually began to follow her lists more closely. Changing the pattern of the evening meal was a greater challenge. Sheila tried buying prepared barbecue chicken, but found the cost too high and the chicken not to her son's taste. The EFNEP aide gave Sheila recipes for broiling and baking chicken, and made sure that she included the necessary ingredients on her shopping list.

Sheila reported that the recipes were difficult to follow, and that both she and Joel preferred their chicken fried. They compromised on an oven-fried recipe that both Sheila and Joel agreed was delicious. Sheila was delighted with her newfound ability to prepare a food that her son enjoyed.

Introducing complex carbohydrates containing essential vitamins and minerals into Joel's diet was an even greater challenge. When left to his own devices, Joel ate sweets—especially his grandmother's baked goods—which were made with lard or shortening. The composition of his original diet, before any of the changes suggested by the aide were introduced, was approximately 12% protein, 48% fat, and 40% carbohydrate, a lot of it simple sugars. The EFNEP aide suggested replacing frozen french fried potatoes with mashed potatoes made with reconstituted skim milk and plain low-fat yogurt. Sheila rejected this idea because she "didn't like yogurt." She did try making mashed potatoes with 2% fat milk and margarine, thereby decreasing the fat intake and increasing protein, vitamin, and mineral content of the meal. Joel loved the mashed potatoes.

The aide arranged her next home visit with Sheila for a time that Joel would be present. She talked with him about his Head Start class and what vegetables he was learning about in his class. The three of them agreed that Sheila would buy some carrots and a vegetable scraper when she shopped next, and Joel would show his mother how he scraped carrots in his Head Start class. Then they would eat the raw carrots with their dinner.

At about this point, Sheila got married. Her husband considered the visits of the EFNEP aide an intrusion into his home and resented it. He said that he could take care of his family and did not want "some government worker telling his wife what to do." Sheila and Joel were lost to the EFNEP program and any subsequent follow-up.

Anna (a Pima tribe Native American)
Joanne Hurley, MS, RD (research dietitian at the Gila River reservation in Arizona)

Anna is 8 1/2 years old. She is 53 in. in height and weighs 150.5 lb. Fifty-six percent of the girls in Anna's second-grade class are above the 95th percentile in weight for height. Anna's story is thus typical of many of her schoolmates.

Anna weighed 7 lb 8 1/2 oz at birth and was 19 1/2 in. long, placing her in the 50th percentile for weight for height. Her mother was not diabetic before or during the pregnancy. She participated in the Women, Infants, and Children (WIC) program, receiving food provided by the program. By the time Anna was 3 months old, she had reached the 90th percentile for weight for height, and by

6 months of age, the 95th percentile. She remained at this level until she reached the age of 2 1/2 when she began to gain weight rapidly.

Anna's mother is a Pima Indian; her father is Hispanic. Anna was the first child born to her mother, who was 18 years of age. Psychosocial factors appear to contribute to Anna's weight gain. She eats to ease her pain of being abandoned by her mother, of being held back a grade in school, of being ridiculed by her peers, and of being cared for most of the time by her maternal grandparents. They feed and care for her, but show little emotional attachment to her. They expressed little if any interest in helping her with her problems at school in general or with her weight problem in particular.

She eats breakfast with her grandparents before the bus takes her to school. She then eats another breakfast and lunch at school. After the bus brings her home in the afternoon, she often snacks on soda pop and chips while she watches television. Extra meals and snacks of around 250 to 285 calories have been a major contributor to her dramatic weight gain over a brief period. Small increases in caloric intake on a consistent basis can have a significant effect on body weight over time.

Anna typifies the emotional poverty of being left alone and being fed as a means of social control, that is, "keeping her out of trouble." She experienced periods of special stress, such as those times when she was sent back to her mother who had abandoned her, or when she was having difficulties at school; these contributed to her pattern of behavior. Food became her immediate source of gratification and solace.

In addition, the current food intake patterns of Anna's community contributed to her problem as well. A study recently completed by the Cleveland Clinic reveals that the community as a whole has a very high intake of fat in their diet. Many of the homemakers cook on hot plates or out of doors, and most of the cooking involves frying. Morbid obesity in very young children in this community is adding to the high number of non–insulin-dependent diabetics under the age of 18 in this population (see Howard et al., 1991; Knowler et al., 1991).

Sabrina (a member of an inner-city African-American family)
Edith Snider, MS

Sabrina and her brother live with their grandmother who is responsible for their care. Sabrina was selected as a control child for an undernourished schoolmate in a study of parental behavior in families of undernourished school children (Karp et al., 1984.) Nine such children were selected as age- and sex-matched controls with measurements for height and arm muscle circumference to meet criteria for good nutritional status. Sabrina was one of two control children who were large (height and arm muscle circumference above the 90th percentile) and moderately obese (triceps fat fold above the 85th percentile).

Sabrina's mother lived around the corner from her mother, Sabrina's grandmother. The children often spent weekends with the grandmother. Sabrina usually spent the whole day at school in the Head Start program in the morning and kindergarten in the afternoon. The family did not receive public assistance and had an income that was $34 per month above the cut-off amount for food stamp eligibility.

The study involved an examination of eating and shopping patterns. Sabrina's family ate together 3 times a day whenever possible. In the winter, the grandmother always prepared a hot breakfast for the children before they left for school. At midday, Sabrina and her brother ate the school lunch. The grandmother planned menus daily and was proud of preparing "good home-cooked meals." She reported that the children had healthy appetites. They were encouraged to try everything that was served at the table. The children were served what they requested and were expected to eat all that they were served. They were not allowed to waste food.

If Sabrina and her brother were hungry between meals, they could go to the kitchen and find snacks to eat. The family would eat out at times or during visits with friends. Sabrina was given pocket money to take with her to school, and she would use it to buy "treats."

One variable that was followed in the study was whether or not families prepared their own food or depended on prepared convenience-food items. A kitchen inventory in Sabrina's grandmother's home revealed that 42% of the food in the home required preparation by an adult (eggs, meat, vegetables); 37% was nutritious convenience food (milk, bread); and 21% was non-nutritious convenience food (soda, chips). The high percentage of food requiring preparation reflected the very structured mealtime pattern in this home. Healthy snack foods were available; the amount of sweet so-called junk food was low.

With respect to the support structure provided to the children, the grandmother's relationship was very positive. Sabrina and her brother were stimulated with books, musical instruments, and various outings. They were taught to be independent and responsible. The character of the family, which was headed by the grandmother, rather than the mother, reveals the importance of the "pivotal person" (see Bradley's comments in chapter 20). The grandmother nurtured the children, although in terms of food intake, the children were probably overfed. Apparently, the family did not consider obesity to be a problem.

Bernard (a member of a Caribbean immigrant family in Brooklyn)
Robert J. Karp, MD

Bernard, age 3, is the youngest of two sons of Mrs. Bonneau, a 28-year-old Haitian woman, who has lived in the United States for 7 years. Bernard and his older brother Andre, age 6, were both born in Brooklyn. Two years ago, as part of routine health care at the Brooklyn Pediatric Resource Center, Andre and his mother were found to have a positive tuberculin test. Bernard was negative. A follow-up chest X-ray showed Mrs.

Bonneau to have active tuberculosis. She was treated with isoniazid and rifampin. Andre, whose chest X-ray was negative, was treated with isoniazid only.

Clinic personnel reassured Mrs. Bonneau that they were not worried about her condition, telling her that she had only a mild illness that is easily treated. But she was not reassured. All she was able to focus on was that "Andre is too skinny; he does not eat."

This attitude that overweight is healthy and being skinny is not was one that was common among Central and Eastern European immigrants who came to the United States in large numbers at the turn of the century. At that time, tuberculosis was the leading cause of death in Europe and in the United States. The disease was associated with wasting, but even Sir Willam Osler, the leading physician in the English-speaking world at that time, was uncertain as to whether the wasting was a cause or consequence of the disease. In his 1889 edition of *The Principles and Practice of Medicine*, Osler gives Hippocrates's description of the "phthitic habitus" of partial emaciation. This appearance was recognized as "too skinny" by Central and Eastern European immigrant grandmothers. Today, in the world's poorest nations, as many as 5 million children per year die in a context of undernutrition. These children are susceptible to chronic infection with gastroenteritis often being the final event before death (see Rabinowitz' comments in chapter 15). Thus, for a child to be too skinny provides a rationale for Mrs. Bonneau to attempt to overfeed her children.

In fact, Andre is a lean child, whereas Bernard has the body shape preferred almost universally by the Caribbean immigrant families, (i.e., slightly overweight) (see Figure 12.2).

Based on comments by Mrs. Bonneau and other Haitian mothers, one could conclude that all Haitian children stop eating when they reach about 1 year of age. The natural diminution in appetite that does occur in all babies nearing their first birthday seems to create panic in these families. "My baby doesn't eat," is the invariable concern. Thus, these immigrant mothers work to get their children to eat and are rewarded by their culture if they are successful as evidenced by the production of slightly to moderately overweight children. This practice contributes to the higher prevalence of obesity in first- and second-generation immigrants (Dietz & Gordon, 1981; Goldblatt et al., 1965) with all of the associated consequences. The task of the clinic professional staff is to encourage these mothers to limit the weight gain of their children, a concept difficult for these mothers to accept, especially if the staff members who are advising them are themselves "too skinny."

The best hope for influencing these familial patterns is that the educational efforts of health professionals will take effect in the next generation when these parents, as grandparents, repeat the advice that they were given. It is clear that very special efforts are needed to prevent obe-

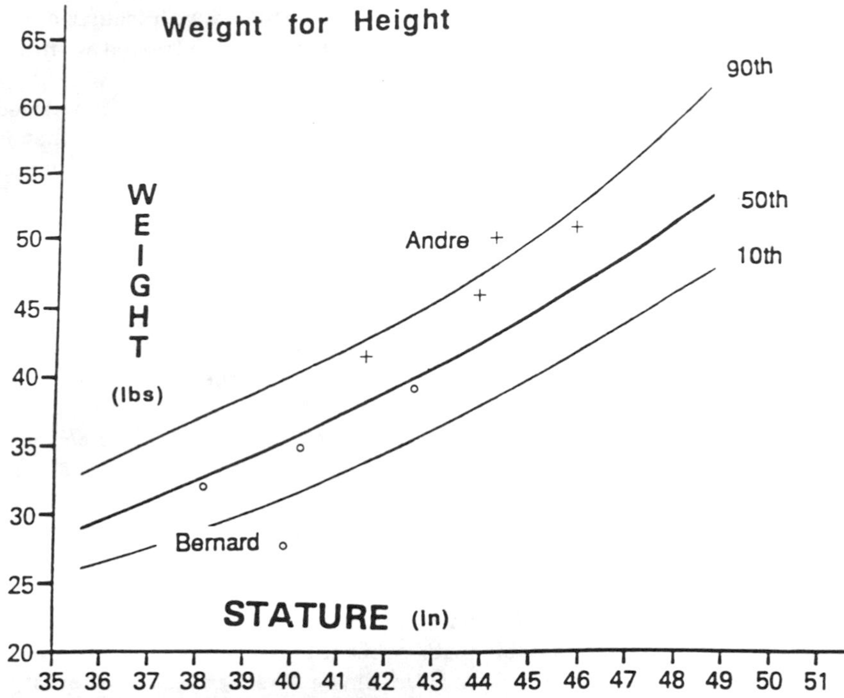

FIGURE 12.2 Weight for height for two young brothers.

sity in the generation of children who arrive with newly immigrant parents from developing countries.

SUMMARY

What lessons can be learned from these case studies of obesity in a variety of familial settings in which poverty, or near poverty, and the development of childhood obesity are the common denominators? Although it is probably the case that all of these situations certainly involve genetic-environmental interactions, environmental stimuli in each of these cases are strongly determinant. In all four cases, the families have easy access to an ample food supply. Thus, although they are poor people in American society, they find themselves far enough away from true poverty that food deprivation is unlikely. Socially determined overeating is likely to occur with this set of circumstances. In each case, an across-generational influence is working; the grandmothers are involved. Although we have no direct data on the matter, we can speculate that the grandmothers bring to the situation memories of familial histories that influence feeding practices. These may take the form of "Eat when food is plentiful against the time when it may not be so." Thus, cultural influences are important factors. These studies are representative of data in the literature, which establish that sociocultural and economic factors exert an early influence on the development of obesity. For example, Stunkard et al. (1972) reported that a population of girls from lower socioeconomic class had an incidence of obesity of 8% compared with 0% for girls from an upper socioeconomic group. Lack of physical activity also appears to be a common factor in these cases. Anna watches television after school; Joel also watches television and helps his grandmother cook; Sabrina is in school most of the day, although she is sometimes taken on "outings." Thus, although overfeeding is a major factor in the development of overweight and obesity in these children from poor families, patterns of inactivity contribute as well. Direct positive correlations between energy expenditure, and body weight and body fat have been reported (Jequier, 1984; Ravussin et al., 1988).

Intervention by professionals to attempt to prevent overweight and obesity from developing in children from families living at the poverty level is a worthy and necessary goal. The patterns established in such children may be continued as they age, setting them up for progressive obesity, which increases their risk of becoming obese adults (National Research Council, 1989) with all of the associated health risks. This is not an easy task, because long established cultural and familial patterns will need to be addressed. Interventions must be appropriately structured to help the parents, grandparents, and children understand the potential long-term sequelae of obesity and the benefits of weight control. For example, long-established familial preferences, particularly in African-American families, for high-fat, fried foods will be contradictory to advice given by health professionals that low-fat diets should be considered (Wadden et al., 1990). The best approach may be an attempt to achieve a few well-defined interventions in patterns related to acquisition and preparation of food of the kind exemplified by the EFNEP aide in the first case study. For example, efforts should be made to decrease the calories derived from fat in the diet to around 30% and encourage the consumption of complex carbohydrates. Activities to increase energy expenditure should be suggested. It is important to remember that a modification of dietary patterns, including modest reduction in food intake, in combination with enhanced physical activity will modulate adiposity in growing children, more so than in adults. Severe food restriction is almost never warranted, and it may lead to negative impacts on linear growth. Some behavioral objectives appropriate for a disadvantaged population could include (a) the improvement of parental shopping and food preparation skills; (b) a reduction in the dependence on saturated fats, such as lard, in food preparation and consumption; an initial approach with respect to consumption might involve encouraging a switch from whole milk (3.5% fat) products to milk products with reduced fat content (2 or 1% fat); (c) introduction of fruits and vegetables into the diet; (d) encouragement of parents and other family members to play active games with their children; (e) discouragement of excessive time spent by children watching television (Dietz & Gortmaker, 1985); (f) in the case of some families, especially those living in rural areas, encouragement of participation by children in activities of gardening, canning, and freezing vegetables.

Clinical experience in the long-term management of obesity indicates that obesity, once established, is difficult to reverse; recidivism rate after weight loss may be as high as 90% (National Research Council, 1989). Thus the best treatment is likely to be prevention. Furthermore, recent studies show that frequent fluctuations in body weight, or weight cycling, are not desirable and may in fact increase risk for chronic disease (Jequier, 1984). Thus, continued efforts by health professionals to intervene to prevent the development of obesity in this population are clearly warranted.

REFERENCES

Bouchard, C. (1989). Genetic factors in obesity. *Medical Clinics of North America, 73*, 67–81.

Bouchard, C., Savard, R., Despres, J. P., et al. (1985). Body composition in adopted and biological siblings. *Human Bio., 57*, 61–75.

Bray, G. A. (Ed.). (1976). *Obesity in perspective: Parts 1 and 2* (Fogarty International Center Series on Preventive Medicine, Vol. 2) Department of Health, Education and Welfare Department Publication No. [NIH] 76–852). Washington, DC.

Callaway, C. W., & Greenwood, M. R. C. (1984). Introduction to the workshop on methods for characterizing human obesity. *Int. J. Obesity*, 477.

Dietz, W. H., & Gordon, J. E. (1981). Obesity in infants, children and adolescents in the United States: II. Causality. *Nutr. Res., 1*, 193–208.

Garn, S. (1986). Family-line and socioeconomic factors in fatness and obesity. *Nutrition Reviews, 44*, 381–386.

Goldblatt, P. B., Moore, M. E., & Stunkard, A. J. (1965). Social factors in obesity. *JAMA, 192*, 97–102.

Gortmaker, S. L., Dietz, W. H., Sobol, A. M., et al. (1987). Increasing pediatric obesity in the United States. *Am J Dis. Child, 141*, 535–540.

Hamm, P. B., Shekelle, R. B., & Stamler, J. (1989). Large fluctuations in body weight during young adulthood and 25-year risk of coronary death in men. *Amer. J. Epidem., 129*, 312–318.

Howard, B. V., Bogardus, C., Ravussin, E., et al. (1991). Studies of the etiology of obesity in Pima Indians. *Am J Clin Nutrition, 53*, 1577S–1585S.

Jequier, E. (1984). Energy expenditure in obesity. *Clin. Endocrinol. Metab., 13*, 563–580.

Karp, R., Nuchpakdee, M., Fairorth, J., & Gorman, J. M. (1976). The school health service as a means of entry into the inner-city family for the identification of malnourished children. *Am. J. Clin. Nutrition, 29*, 216–218.

Karp, R. J., Scholl, T. O., Decker, D., & Ebert, E. (1989). Growth of abused children contrasted with the non-abused in an urban poor community. *Clin. Pediatrics, 28*, 317–320.

Karp, R. J., Snider, E., Fairorth, J. W., et al. (1984). Parental behavior and the availability of foods among undernourished inner-city school children. *J. Fam. Prac., 18*, 731–35.

Knowler, W. C., Pettitt, D. J., Saad, M. F., et al. (1991). Obesity in the Pima Indians: Its magnitude and relationship with diabetes. *Am J Clin Nutr, 53*, 1543S–1551S.

Lapidus, L., Andersso, H., Bengtsson, C., & Bosaeus, I. (1986). Dietary habits in relation to incidence of cardiovascular disease and death in women: A 12-year follow-up of participants in the population study of women in Gothenburg, Sweden. *Am. J. Clin. Nutr., 44*, 444–448.

National Research Council of the National Academy of Sciences. (1989). Diet and health report: Implications for reducing chronic disease risk. Washington, DC: National Academy Press.

Price, R. A., Cadoret, R. J., Stunkard, A. J., & Troughton, E. (1987). Genetic contributions to human fatness: An adoption study. *Am. J. Psychiatry, 144*, 1003–1008.

Ravussin, E., Lillioja, S., Knowler, W. C., et al. (1988). Reduced rate of energy expenditure as a risk factor for body-weight gain. *N. Engl. J. Med., 318*, 467–472.

Rimm, A. A., & White, P. L. (1979). Obesity: Its risks and hazards. In G. Bray (Ed.), *Obesity in America* (NIH Publication No. 79–359). Washington, DC: U.S. Department of Health, Education and Welfare.

Sorensen, T. T. A., Price, R. A., Stunkard, A. J., & Schulsinger, F. (1988). Genetics of obesity in adult adoptees and their biological siblings. *Br. Med. J., 298*, 87–90.

Stunkard, A. J., D'Aquili, E., Fox, S., & Filion, R. D. L. (1972). The influence of social class on obesity and thinness in children. *J. Am. Med. Assn., 22*, 579–584.

Stunkard, A. J., Sorensen, T., Hanis, C., et al. (1986). An adoption study of human obesity. *N. Engl. J. Med., 314*, 193–198.

U.S. Department of Health and Human Services. (1988). *The Surgeon General's report on nutrition and health* (DHHS Publication No. 88–50210). Washington, DC: U.S. Government Printing Office.

Van Itallie, T. B. (1985). Health implications of overweight and obesity in the United States. *Annals of Internal Medicine, 103*, 983–988.

Wachs, E. D., & Gruen, G. (1982). *Early experience and human development.* New York: Plenum.

Wadden, T. A., Stunkard, A. J., Rich, L., et al. (1990). Obesity in black adolescent girls: A controlled clinical trial of treatment by diet, behavior modification and parental support. *Pediatrics, 85*, 345–352.

13

Prevention of Hypertension

Julie R. Ingelfinger, MD

Hypertension is, in general, a silent problem in children and adolescents. Significant morbidity and mortality occur with persistent, severe elevation of blood pressure in adults. Though severe hypertension in childhood is also associated with serious morbidity and mortality (Lloyd-Still, 1967), the major concern for this chapter is prevention of the mild blood pressure elevation that starts in childhood since even mild hypertension places adults, both male and female, at risk.

The relationship between poverty and rates of hypertension is a complex one. The rate of hypertension is consistently higher among black as compared with white populations (Dridz et al., 1986). But the concern here is not simply that there is a concomitant increase in the proportion of poor people who are black, but that the poor of all ethnic and racial backgrounds are less likely to get the careful medical supervision required to provide sound dietary advice and treat hypertension.

To be addressed in this chapter are the key elements in a preventive program including the relationship between heredity and environment and the elements of a preventive program. Discussions of other issues of importance that are beyond the scope of this text (including the physiology of blood pressure control and the process of screening for hypertension) can be found in Ingelfinger (1989, 1990) and Horan et al. (1987).

PHENOMENON OF "TRACKING"

One approach is to study the tendency toward hypertension (rather than occurrence) by means of tracking, for example, the tendency of individuals at a given percentile of the distribution of blood pressure level to remain at that percentile as they grow older (Lauer et al., 1984). The concept of tracking provides the best predictor presently available to determine future risk. For example, a boy with a blood pressure of 107/69 mmHg at age 5 years and 118/74 mmHg at age 10 years is tracking along the 90th percentile for his age. For reference, Figure 13.1 shows nomograms from the Second Task Force on Blood Pressure Control in Children for blood pressure for children from ages 2 to 18 (Horan et al., 1987).

HEREDITY, NUTRITION, AND RISK FOR HYPERTENSION

The foods we eat, the nutrients contained within our diets and the relationships among various dietary minerals such as sodium, potassium, calcium, and magnesium have a profound effect on measures of blood pressure (McCarron et al., 1984; Tobian, 1988). As is shown in chapter 19 on diets of poorer ethnic groups, the dietary characteristics of disadvantaged children are, unfortunately, similar to those that make a child prone to hypertension latter in life—excess sodium, decreased potassium, calcium and magnesium.

A high percentage of the adult American population is hypertensive. Of individuals with primary hypertension (the bulk of these with elevated blood pressure) there is frequently a strong family history of elevated blood pressure. About half of these individuals with primary hypertension appear salt sensitive—that is blood pressure goes up with increased salt intake. Several cross-cultural studies have demonstrated that blood pressure varies directly with sodium chloride intake, at least at the extremes of reported dietary intakes. A very high salt intake (as in northern Japan) or very low salt intake (as in Eskimo society) is associated, respectively, with high and low blood pressure when one looks at the communities as a whole (Dahl, 1977). Associating a midrange of salt intake with blood pressure level is more

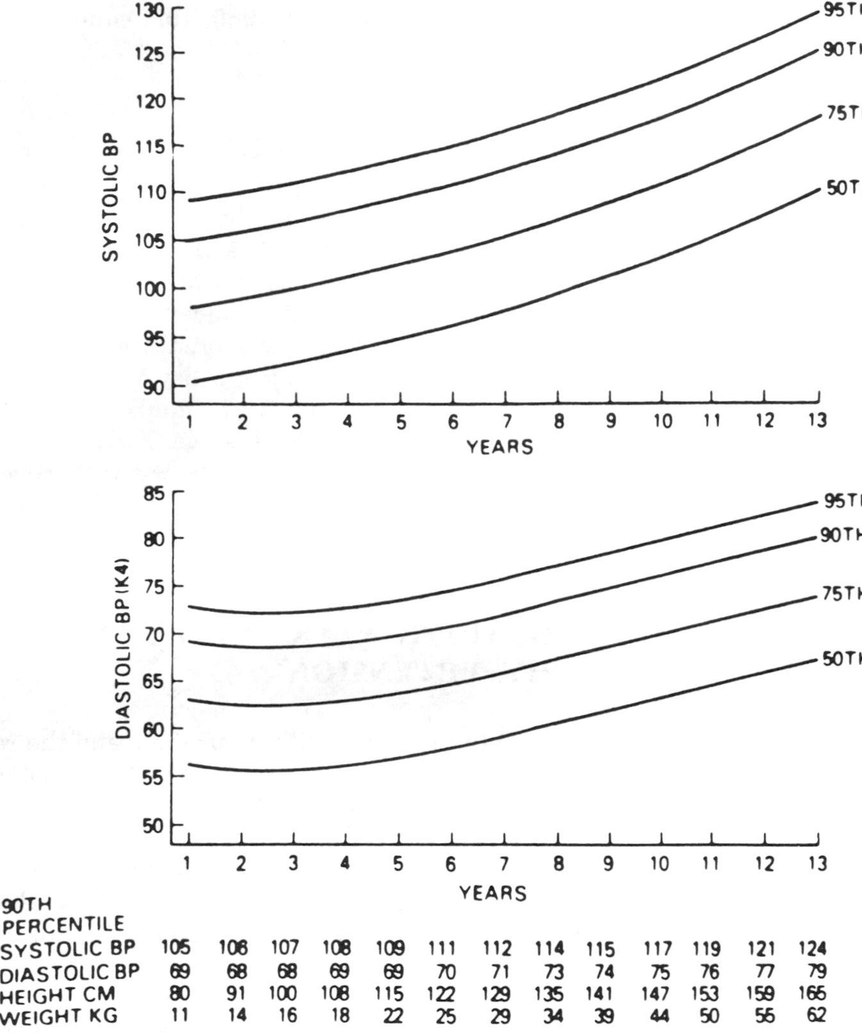

90TH PERCENTILE													
SYSTOLIC BP	105	106	107	108	109	111	112	114	115	117	119	121	124
DIASTOLIC BP	69	68	68	69	69	70	71	73	74	75	76	77	79
HEIGHT CM	80	91	100	108	115	122	129	135	141	147	153	159	165
WEIGHT KG	11	14	16	18	22	25	29	34	39	44	50	56	62

FIGURE 13.1 Normative data from the Second Task Force on Blood Pressure Control in Children—1987. Normal Blood Pressure for boys ages 1–13 are shown.

From Horan et al. (1987).

problematic. Salt intake is determined by habit, and this may obscure the phenomenon of salt sensitivity. Salt intake is only important in those individuals who are salt sensitive.

When considering dietary salt intake and its implication for health care, the Second Task Force on Blood Pressure Control in Children stated:

> It is apparent that the sodium intake of children is far in excess of that required for optimal growth and development. Thus the potential benefit of dietary salt reduction in hypertension appears to outweigh any potential risk from this form of therapy. (Horan et al., 1987)

It is difficult to predict which children with family histories of hypertension will develop elevated blood pressure. Many youngsters will not respond to salt intake with an elevation in blood pressure, but a family history showing one parent with salt-sensitive hypertension is suggestive that the patient may also develop the condition. Among American population groups, black Americans seem to have the highest risk of salt-sensitive hypertension. The dietary contribution to this problem is discussed in chapters 18 and 19.

Mineral Nutrients

At the highest and lowest amounts of dietary sodium chloride intake in a given community, blood pressure within the population seems to correlate directly. However, in the midrange of salt intake within a given community's association between salt and blood pressure is less clear. By contrast, potassium, calcium, and magnesium intake appears to be correlated inversely with blood pressure.

Renal Function

It has been suggested that in normal individuals, there is an increase in salt intake that leads to increased extracellular fluid volume. The kidney is stimulated to increase urine output and to turn off renin release and adrenal response to angiotensin II (mediators of salt and water retention) (Shoback et al., 1983). In a low-salt state the reverse would occur. Some individuals with primary hypertension who fail to make this modulation quickly enough develop a new, elevated setpoint for blood pressure.

Obesity

As noted in the preceding chapter, obesity has been associated with blood pressure elevation for some time (Reisin et al., 1978; Rocchini et al., 1986). One reason for the association is that indirect measurement of blood pressure is obtained first by occluding the artery over which pressure is to be measured with a cuff that encircles the arm. Systolic pressure, or Korotokoff 1 (Kl), is taken as the signal or sound generated when blood begins to flow through the artery as the occluding pressure is gradually lowered or released. Too small a blood pressure cuff requires an artificially high "pressure" to compress the vessel and may artifactually cause "hypertension." However, truly higher blood pressure levels and frank hypertension do appear to be associated with obesity in some patients.

PREVENTION AND DIET THERAPY

Children who have severe blood pressure elevation require drug therapy (Horan et al., 1987). Nonpharmacological therapies are optimal for mild hypertension in childhood. The following set of guidelines is intended for use in youngsters with mild blood pressure elevation. The dietary guidelines are pragmatic and suggested with the thought that approximately half of individuals with hypertension are salt sensitive.

Nonpharmacological therapy should involve weight reduction to optimal levels, life-style change with more aerobic exercise, and dietary adjustment. Clearly, whether such an approach is effective is related both to the educational success of explaining the program, the reinforcement on the part of the health care professional, and the motivation on the part of the patient and his or her family. Weight-loss programs for young children should involve the entire family. Exercise and peer-group activities are encouraged for overweight teens. Not only does aerobic exercise lead to a decrease in blood pressure but appears to have a beneficial effect on plasma lipids. While weight training (isometric exercises) will reduce resting blood pressure, it has a questionable effect on cardiovascular fitness and is not generally recommended. Before participation in organized sports, a youngster with marked blood pressure elevation should be evaluated with an echocardiogram, as well as exercise testing. Children with an undue pressor response to exercise should have pharmacological as well as nonpharmacological therapy.

No child or adult should be asked to go on a no-added–salt diet when blood pressure elevation is first detected. This guarantees "no compliance" rather than "no salt." Fortunately, as Beauchamp has shown (1987), a stepwise approach can be successful, and a coating of foods with a small amount of sodium after preparation has the same salty flavor (Beachamp et al., 1990). Fortunately, it would appear that there is more general awareness in the population concerning nutritionally sound foods. The availability of no-added–salt foods with no extra cost would be especially efficacious.

SUMMARY

In general, the youngster at risk for developing hypertension is overweight with a family history of either primary hypertension or hypertension-associated systemic diseases (e.g., neurofibromatosis). Because the appetite for particular foods takes months, if not longer to change, an at-risk youngster is encouraged to have a relatively low-salt diet and polyunsaturated-fat diet from a young age. The inclusion of fresh fruits and vegetables with their high potassium to sodium ratio as well as low-fat milk products with added calcium also are encouraged as preventive measures.

Education is the mainstay of nonpharmacological therapy for hypertension. But it is difficult to obtain dietary compliance because change is requested for an asymptomatic condition. Thus, all of the following should be discussed with the family:

1. Concept of cardiovascular risk factors
2. Implications of a family history of hypertension and hyperlipidemias
3. Effects of tobacco and alcohol in cardiovascular disease (alcohol and tobacco use, in any case, should be discouraged in children and adolescents)
4. Importance of remaining lean and active

Change in diet, in addition to weight loss, has focused on decreasing sodium and increasing potassium intake. It is unnecessary to restrict salt intake severely, as moderate reductions are often quite effective. Recommending good foods and acceptable levels of salt intake are more helpful than providing a list of "don't eat this, don't eat that," which has characterized much dietary counseling. Chapter 19 presents positive ways of encouraging healthful eating habits as does the next chapter with a discussion of the prudent diet.

REFERENCES

Beauchamp, G. (1987). The human preference for excess salt. *American Scientist, 75*, 27–33.

Beauchamp, G. K., Bertino, M., Burke, D., & Engelman, K. (1990). Experimental sodium depletion and salt taste in normal human volunteers. *Am J Clin Nutrition, 51*, 881–890.

Dahl, L. K. (1977). Salt intake and hypertension. In J. Genest, O. Kuchel, P. Hamet, and M. Cantin, (Eds.), *Hypertension* (2nd ed., pp. 548–59). New York: McGraw-Hill.

Dahl, L. K., & Love, R. M. (1954). Evidence of relationship between sodium (chloride) intake and human hypertension. *Arch. Intern Med., 94*, 525–531.

Drizd, T., et al. (1986). Blood pressure levels in persons 18–74 years of age (U.S. National Health Survey, Series 11, No. 234). Hyattsville, MD: U.S. Public Health Service.

Horan, M. J., Blaustein, M. P., Dunbar, J. H., et al. (1985). NIH report on research challenges in nutrition and hypertension. *Hypertension, 7*, 818–823.

Ingelfinger, J. (1989). Nutritional aspects of pediatric hypertension. *Bull NY Acad Med, 65*, 1109–1120.

Ingelfinger, J. (1990). Hypertension and renovascular disease. *Pediatric Annals, 2*, 343–347.

Lauer, R. M., Anderson, A. R., Beaglehole, R., et al. (1984). Factors related to tracking of blood pressure in children: U.S. National Center for Health Statistics Health Examination Surveys, Cycles II and III. *Hypertension, 6*, 307.

Lloyd-Still, J., & Cottom, D. G. (1967). Severe hypertension in childhood. *Arch Dis Child, 42*, 34–39.

McCarron, D. A., Morris, C. D., Henry, J. H., et al. (1984). Blood pressure and nutrient intake in the United States. *Science, 224*, 1392–1398.

Reisin, E. D., Abel, R., Modan, M. (1978). Effect of weight loss without salt restriction on the reduction of blood pressure in overweight hypertensive patients. *N Engl J Med, 298*, 1–6.

Rocchini, A. P., Katch, V. L., Grekin, R., et al. (1986). Role for aldosterone in blood pressure regulation of obese adolescents. *Am J Cardiol, 57*, 613–618.

Shoback, D. M., Williams, G. H., & Moore, T. J., et al. (1983). Defect in the sodium modulated tissue responsiveness to angiotensin II in essential hypertension. *J Clin Invest, 72*, 2115-2124.

Tobian, L. (1988). Potassium and hypertension. *Nutrition Reviews, 46*, 273–283.

14

Prevention of Coronary Heart Disease Among Disadvantaged Children

Robert J. Karp, MD, Marilyn Winkleby, PhD, Andrew Bostom, MD, and Stephen Wadowski, MD

Many of the risk factors for coronary heart disease (CHD) in adults have their origins in infancy and childhood. The need, therefore, is to identify those children who are at risk for CHD later in life. The question is: How? Devising strategies to prevent CHD is difficult for adults and even more so for children (Barness, 1986; McNamara, 1986).

Data examining the relationship between premorbid cardiovascular disease risk factors and the development of overt CHD have been derived from predominantly adult white male populations (Levy et al., 1990; Stamler et al., 1986). In general, these studies have included too few, nonwhite minority individuals for meaningful comparisons. Prospective epidemiological investigations of large adult minority populations have begun recently. Only preliminary data are available for addressing the question of whether risk factors for CHD are the same in white and minority populations. Furthermore, studies are only beginning to examine the degree to which poverty explains racial differences in CHD risk factors.

In this chapter we consider racial and income differences in the occurrence of CHD, examine interaction of risk factors, and suggest development of appropriate preventive strategies. Although the incidence of CHD rose to epidemic proportions to become the leading cause of adult death in this century, there has been a striking decline in CHD mortality since about 1968 (Goldman, 1990). To understand this phenomenon and to ensure a continuing fall in death rates requires a consideration of the pathogenesis of CHD. As related to future trends for children, we need to learn effective interventions for youth, especially those from high risk disadvantaged homes, so that rates of CHD in adult life can be lessened.

RISK FACTORS FOR CHD

The three major modifiable risk factors for CHD are hypercholesterolemia, cigarette smoking, and hypertension, with smoking and hypertension the most likely to affect the lives of children who are black, poor, and of limited education (Levy et al., 1990). Identifying the first factor, hypercholesterolemia, is the most problematic because, under usual circumstances, the identification of mild to moderate hypercholesterolemia requires no more treatment than the "prudent diet" recommended to all children.

With respect to these three factors, the pediatric and adult medical communities agree that prevention of smoking and better education about all the risk factors are essential. Children and adolescents should be encouraged to maintain a prudent diet with regular exercise and avoidance of smoking. Unfortunately, among disadvantaged children, the availability of nutritious food or even a safe place to exercise may be lacking.

Racial and Income Differences

During the last decade racial disparities in rates of coronary heart disease have been documented for black as compared with white adults living in the United States. Epidemiological studies of CHD present a relatively consistent picture, with blacks experiencing higher rates than whites for both sexes and in most age groups. Although consistent results have emerged, few studies have examined the extent to which socioeconomic status confounds the racial differences in CHD. Furthermore, few studies have compared rates in whites with other minority groups in the United States.

One inconsistency has arisen from clinical reports of CHD mortality in blacks and whites that suggest that fatal CHD is lower for blacks than for whites. Examination of death rates from CHD over the last 30 years, however, show that this impression is inaccurate. Increases in rates of CHD among blacks during the 1950s and 1960s resulted in similar rates for black and white males, and higher rates for black than white females (Gillum et al., 1984). During the 1980s, declines in cases of fatal CHD leveled off for black males as well as black females (Sempose et al., 1988), causing higher mortality rates for black males until age 65 and black females until age 75 when compared with whites. Currently, blacks consistently exhibit higher rates of fatal CHD than whites in all age groups after age 15, with the magnitude of the differences being approximately twofold. Larger differences are shown between black and white adults for fatal cases of hypertension and hypertensive heart disease, with blacks showing rates up to 6 times higher than whites (Vital Statistics, 1988). Although the mechanisms that explain the black-white differences in mortality are unclear, it appears that differences in prevalence of hypertension may account for much of the persistent black-white differences in CHD-related deaths. For instance, the Evans County prospective study of black and white women showed that there was little or no excess risk of CHD deaths among black women after adjustment for blood pressure and level of income (Johnson et al., 1986). In addition to experiencing excess mortality from CHD, blacks in the United States also show higher rates of hypertension and smoking, but findings are inconsistent for hypercholesterolemia. Higher cholesterol subfractions (especially high density lipoprotein), however, have been reported in some community-based studies for black males, including both adults and children (Glueck et al., 1984).

Hypertension

The CHD risk factor with the largest and most consistent black-white difference is for hypertension (Dridz, et al., 1986). This excess risk in African-Americans remains, after adjustment for education, a marker of social class. Unlike adults, ethnic differences in blood pressure among white, black, and Hispanic children in the United States do not show consistent differences (Schacter et al., 1984); however, by adolescence, black children appear to have slightly higher blood pressure than white children (Prineas & Gillum, 1985).

Cigarette Smoking

The excess risk of hypertension among black adults extends to rates of cigarette smoking, but is of a lower magnitude (MMWR, 1987). While rates of smoking among Hispanics in the United States originally appeared to be lower than among whites (especially for Hispanic women), recent evidence suggests the number of cigarettes smoked is higher (Marcus & Crane, 1985). Some studies indicate that rates of smoking among Hispanic school children are higher than among white school children (Greenberg et al., 1987). Smoking rates escalate sharply among all groups of teenagers with the onset in junior high school (Miller & Slap, 1988).

Confounding Effect of Social Class

Because there is clearly a confounding effect of poverty on race, studies need to take socioeconomic status into account when interpreting racial differences in rates of CHD. It is well documented that poverty level differs by race; for example, data from the 1980 census show that 30% of blacks and 24% of Hispanics live below the poverty line as compared with 9% of whites. Although few studies on racial differences in CHD have investigated whether race is independent of poverty status, there is some evidence that racial differences are at least partially attenuated when socioeconomic status is taken into account (Winkleby et al., 1988).

Risk Factor Interaction

Prospective epidemiologic data from both the Framingham Study (Kannel, 1981) and the Multiple Risk Factor Intervention Trial (MRFIT) (Stamler et al., 1986) provide persuasive evidence that CHD risk is substantially increased when the three major CHD risk factors are present in combination. As shown in Figure 14.1, at each quintile of serum total cholesterol in the MRFIT study, concomitant hypertension (diastolic blood pressure > 90 mm Hg) and smoking caused at least a 3.5-increase in CHD mortality, with those in the third and fourth quintile experiencing an approximately 6-fold or greater increase in CHD mortality (Stamler et al., 1986).

Furthermore, as shown in Figures 14.2 and 14.3, cigarette smoking is found disproportionately among those who are least educated and from the lowest income subgroups (i.e., the disadvantaged). Recent work by Winkleby et al. (1990) has shown an inverse relationship between education level and six risk factors for health including the three associated with CHD. Taking advantage of this segment of the population, the major tobacco companies have targeted two groups of

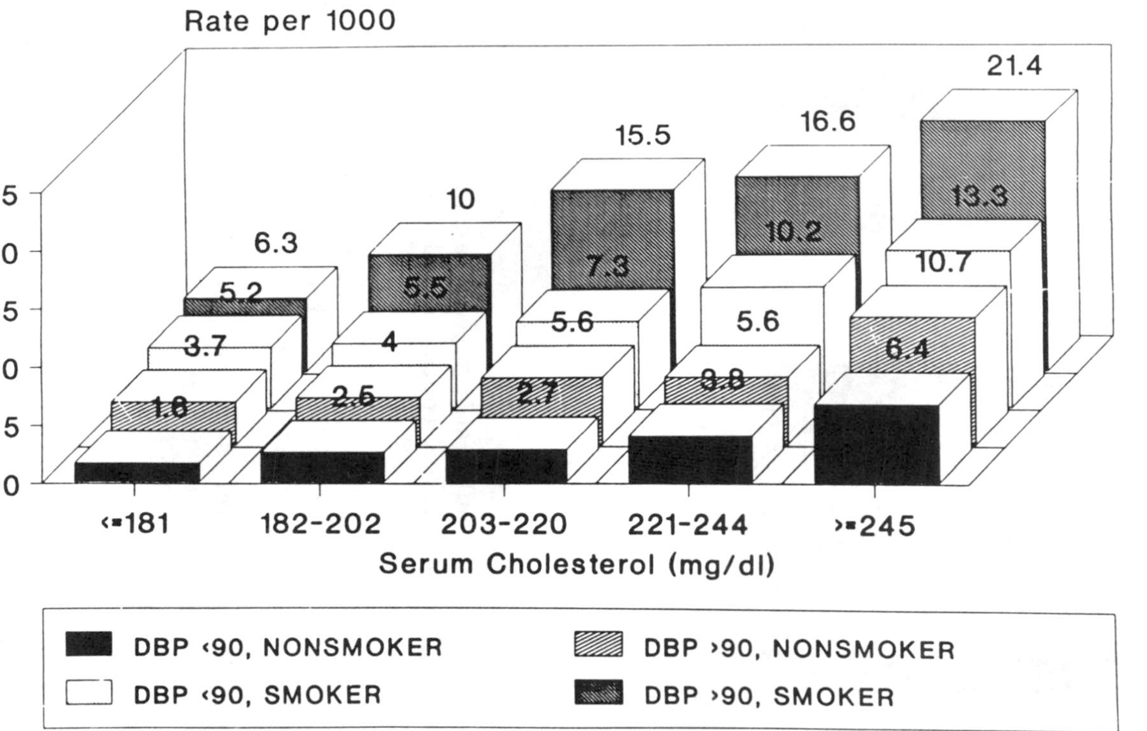

FIGURE 14.1 Relationship of quintiles of serum cholesterol with smoking and diastolic blood pressure elevations as predictors of 6-year coronary heart disease mortality.

From the Multiple Risk Factor Intervention Trial (Stamler et al., 1986).

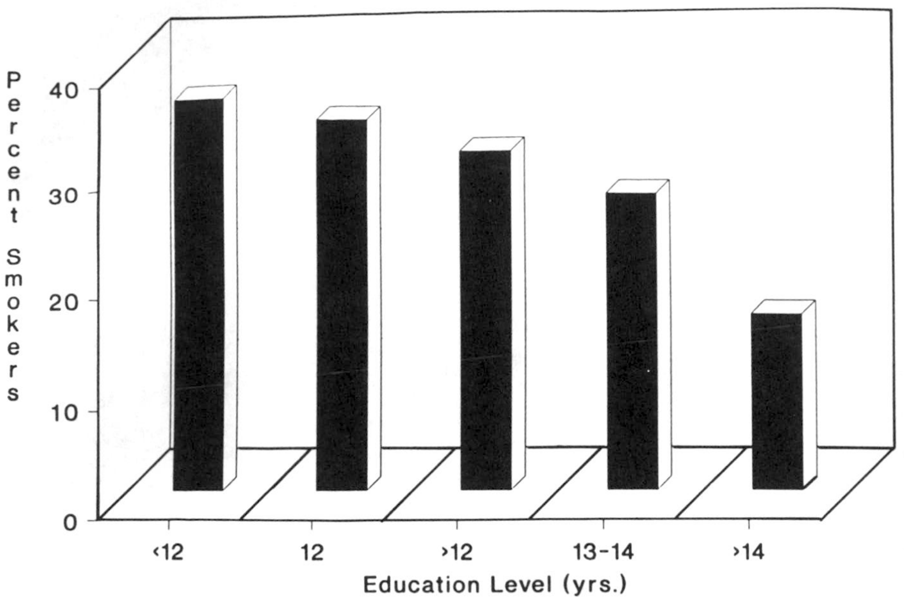

FIGURE 14.2 Education level versus percent of smokers.

From the Centers for Disease Control (*New York Times*, February 24, 1990, Section 4, p. 4).

young people who are most vulnerable to peer pressure and advertising—working women with limited education and black populations (Tuckson, 1989).

HYPERCHOLESTEROLEMIA—CHD THEORY AS RELATED TO CHILDREN

There is an extensive literature supporting claims that elevated serum cholesterol levels predispose to CHD (Grundy, 1986; Stamler et al., 1986). A full discussion of this theory is beyond the scope or intention of this text. Though the theory has become generally accepted, strong, and at times vituperative, critiques have appeared in both the lay (Moore, 1989) and professional press (Brett, 1989). These criticisms are a reasonable response to exaggerated claims. They do not, however, impeach the theory as a mechanism leading to overt clinical pathology in persons affected by multiple risk factors.

The pediatric community has concerns based on the fear that indiscriminate following of the cholesterol-heart theory and the limita-

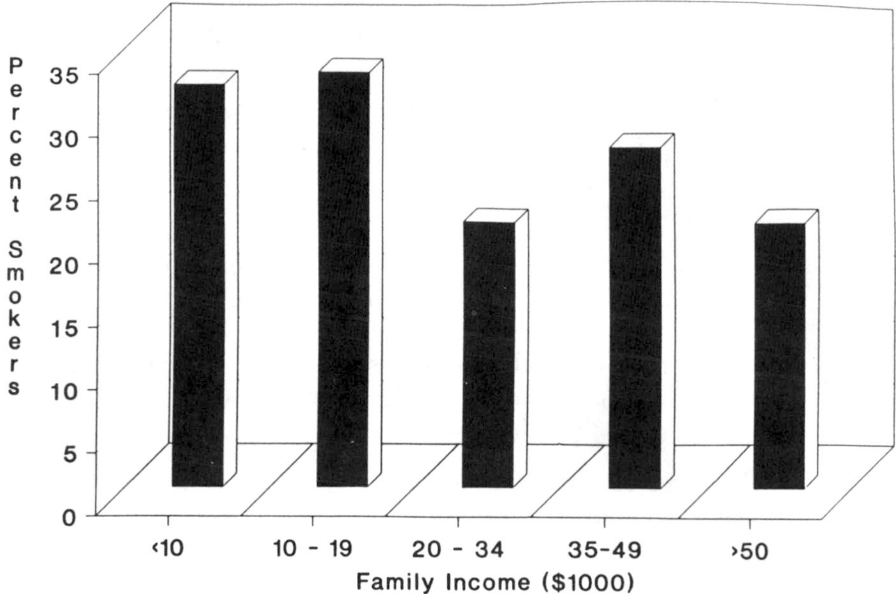

FIGURE 14.3 Family income versus percent smokers.

From the Centers for Disease Control (*New York Times*, February 24, 1990, Section 4, p. 4).

tions it implies will have deleterious effects (McNamara, 1986). Infant diets are generally high in total fat—40% to 50% of calories from fat—a circumstance that appears to be biologically sound during this period of very rapid growth, limited capacity for high volume of food intake, and a need for lipid for a developing nervous system (American Academy of Pediatrics, 1986). This high concentration of fat in the diet is necessary until age 2 years, at the very least. Even past the age of 2 years, the 30% of calories from fat used as a recommended figure for adults must be considered a minimum figure for children. Among young children, excessive zeal applied to the limitation of fat in the diet creates a potential for loss of minerals, especially zinc, iron and calcium, from nutritious high-fat foods. Lifshitz and Moses (1988) have shown growth failure among children placed on imprudent diets because of a "fear of fatness."

For one group of children, however, early intervention is justified with little hesitancy. These are the children (from 1/200 to 1/500 of the population) who have familial hypercholesterolemia (Kwiterovich,

1989) with an additional group of 3% to 5% of children who have polygenic lipid abnormalities influenced by diet as well as heredity.

STRATEGIES TO BE USED FOR SCREENING DISADVANTAGED CHILDREN

Consider three stategies:

1. *Population.* A cholesterol level is measured on children with a positive family history, and all families are given the same advice for a prudent diet and life-style.
2. *Mass screening.* All children have serum cholesterol measured.
3. *Public health.* No screening is suggested because all families are advised for a prudent diet and life-style.

Data collected from 300 of Brooklyn's most disadvantaged children suggest that a population strategy is an appropriate middle ground (Wadowski et al., 1991). For 88 children with a positive history of CHD in parents or grandparents less than 55 years of age, the mean serum cholesterol of 173 mg/dl $\pm$ 38, whereas for the remainder (those without a family history) the mean serum cholesterol was 161 mg/dl $\pm$ 30. These values are significantly different from each other ($p < .005$), but neither the difference in serum cholesterol levels nor the absolute values were unexpected when compared with national samples (Frierichs et al., 1976; Lauer et al., 1988). More important, we found almost 40% of children with a positive family history to have serum cholesterol that was elevated ($>$180 mg/dl). This is a substantially higher positive predictive value for positive family history than has been found in multiple large studies of middle- and upper-income Americans. The data suggest that there is a greater incidence of CHD at a young age among adults in this community with the cause likely to be the concomitant harmful effects of smoking and untreated hypertension (see Figures 14.1 to 14.3).

A pure public health approach would fail to recognize the high percentage of children with both positive family history and elevation in serum cholesterol, and the yield for children with a completely negative history (20% to 25%) was too low to warrant mass screening. A population strategy does maintain the one strength of the public health approach—all children over 2 years age receive the prudent diet.

Mass screening has another drawback. In communities that encounter the social and political diseases of poverty, drugs, crime, disrupted families, and lack of education, the significance of a healthy child's serum cholesterol level may seem relatively unimportant to a parent. As a result the ability to follow up and intervene appropriately when an elevated cholesterol level is discovered in a child is tremendously hindered. Moreover, there is an inherent blindness in policies for screening and prevention that focus so narrowly on serum lipids. Equal attention should be directed at the other risk factors and the interventions needed to improve the level of knowledge and to change behavior in the community.

STRATEGIES FOR PREVENTION

The black-white disparities in CHD argue for primary and secondary prevention programs for black and possibly other minority populations. Primary prevention programs should cover diet, physical fitness, smoking, and blood pressure education. Secondary prevention programs should include early detection and effective treatment of hypertension, weight reduction, and diet modification.

Preventive efforts that address racial and socioeconomic status differences in CHD mortality and risk factors must consider a combination of personal, life-style, environmental, and genetic factors. In addition to these, factors relating to health (e.g., exposure to health information, access to preventive health services), and culture (e.g., attitudes about weight, exercise, medication) must be addressed. When targeting low-income and minority groups, efforts should (a) view prevention as a process to be shared by various levels within society and (b) evaluate factors in the environment that contribute to disease (Wallack & Winkleby, 1987). Consider the billboard in Figure 14.4 that engages the interest of children on their way to the Pratt-Arnold School in Philadelphia. These advertisements remind young children of the desirability of the two products most likely to cut short the lives of young black people, cigarettes and alcohol.

Such advertising has no place in a community concerned about the long-term health of its youth. CHD prevention and other health promotion programs applied to communities rather than to high-risk individuals may be effective with children and adults from the disadvantaged groups who are missed by more traditional models (Farquhar et al., 1990).

Coronary heart disease is a complex, multifactorial disease causing a great deal of morbidity and mortality in the United States. Our "modern lifestyle," which begins in youth, and includes cigarette smoking, a rich diet, and sedentary habits—all of which are risk factors for cardiovascular disease later in life. It is essential, therefore,

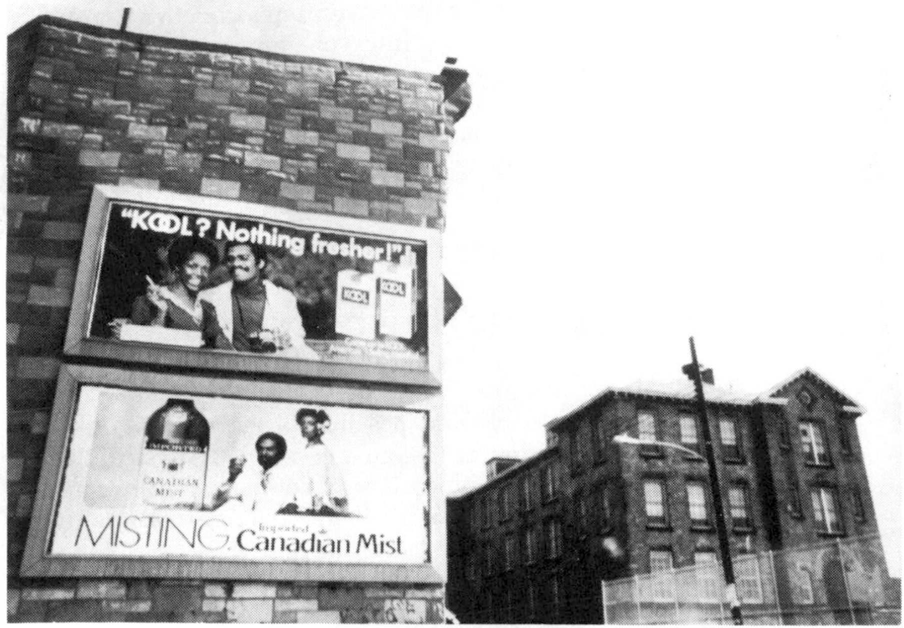

FIGURE 14.4 A billboard advertising cigarettes and alcohol seen by children every day as they walk to school and back home.

Photograph by Leah Jaynes Karp.

that preventive measures target young children at the age when high-risk behaviors are formed. It is most important, especially in the disadvantaged population, to target all risk factors for CHD for intervention including tobacco use, hypertension, obesity, and sedentary life-style as well as serum cholesterol levels.

A Prudent Diet
Carl Senft, MS, and Rene Murray-Bachmann, RD

Although it may seem simple to recommend a prudent diet, changing a person's diet is a very difficult process that includes the constant repetition of simple facts, rebuttal of faddist theories, and slow steps to change. Chapter 19 on the role of ethnicity discusses the nature of dietary advice more fully. What people choose to eat is influenced by taste, flavor, and palatability as well as other factors such as convenience and cost. The employment of any one of these factors as a basis for diet selection can lead the individual to nutritional excess detrimental to long-term health and is one of the greatest stumbling blocks to following a prudent diet.

Even those individuals aware of the impact of diet on their health often seek solution by excess—finding a singular miracle component that

TABLE 14.1 Characteristics of Prudent Diet

Calories	sufficient to maintain lean body weight
Fat	30% of total calories with 1 part saturated to 1 part monounsaturated to 1 part polyunsaturated
Cholesterol	300 mg a day
Carbohydrate	55% of total calories, 45% as long chain polysaccharides. Only 10% of total calories as simple sugars.
Protein	between 12-15% of total calories from mixed sources of dairy products, legumes, and lean meats.
Fiber	emphasis on whole grain cereals and bulky vegetables
Salt	limited to 5 mg NaCl per day from all sources

will purge the body of unwanted toxins (Alhadeff et al., 1984). Publicity given to a few isolated studies resulted in stampedes to the supermarkets and drugstores for grapefruit pectin, oat bran, and fish oil.

Table 14.1 displays the basic content of the prudent diet (Bierman & Chait, 1988).

What changes are needed for Americans to follow the prudent diet? It is recommended that the 600 mg of cholesterol consumed daily be decreased to 300 mg/day and that fat intake currently averaging 43% of their total caloric intake be reduced to 30%—10% as saturated fat, 10% as monounsaturated fat, and 10% as polyunsaturated fat. These changes in cholesterol and fat intake can be implemented by decreasing the consumption of high-fat animal products such as whole milk, cheese, butter, beef, pork, and lard. The caloric deficit associated with this reduction can be made up by increasing sources of complex carbohydrates such as vegetables, fruits, and legumes from an average of 46% to 55%. For many people, the caloric deficit promotes health by helping them to achieve lean body weight. Furthermore, complex carbohydrates from whole-grain cereals and bulky vegetables increase the intake of dietary fiber.

Lower-fat sources of protein, such as fish, poultry, legumes, low-fat dairy products and lean cuts of meat should be encouraged. Currently, Americans derive 12% of their total calories from protein that is probably satisfactory. The idea that protein-containing foods are "better" than carbohydrates increases the cost of food for the poor unnecessarily.

How achievable is a prudent diet for the poor? In fact, when families have the resources and ability to prepare food, the traditional fare of poorer people is nutritious and can be quite prudent, but the constraints on poor families are different from those on the more affluent. The comment of Margaret Mead that food habits of the affluent "sift down as 'style' to the lower income levels" seems appropriate here (1943). Cost does matter. For example, olive oil, which is rich in monounsaturates, is substantially more expensive than other liquid fats. For another example, urban poor families are unlikely to have an inexpensive source of fresh vegetables or fruit. Lean cuts of beef and pork, when considered on a per-calorie basis, are more expensive than fatty ones, but the use of smaller portions of lean meat provides better nutrition at no additional cost.-

REFERENCES

Aldaheff, L., Gualteri, T., & Lipton, M. (1984). Toxic effects of water soluble vitamins. *Nut Rev, 42*, 33–40.

American Academy of Pediatrics, Committee on Nutrition. (1986). Prudent life-style for children: Dietary fat and cholesterol. *Pediatrics, 78*, 521–525.

Barness, L. A. (1986). Cholesterol and children. *JAMA, 256*, 2871.

Bierman, E. L., & Chait, A. (1989). In M. E. Shils, & V. Young (Eds.), *Modern nutrition in health and disease*, (6th ed., pp. 1283–1297). Philadelphia: Lea & Febiger.

Brett, A. S. (1989). Treating hypercholesterolemia: how should practising physicians interpret the published data for patients. *NEJM, 321*, 679–680.

Drizd, T., Dannenberg, A. L., & Engel, A. (1986). Blood pressure levels in persons 18–74 years of age (Data from the U.S. National Health Survey, Series 11, No. 234). Hyattsville, MD: U.S. Public Health Service.

Farquhar, J. W., Fortmann, S. P., Flora, J. A., et al. (1990). Effects of community-wide education on cardiovascular disease risk factors: The Stanford Five-City Project. *JAMA, 264*, 359–365.

Gillum, R. F., Liuy, K. C., et al. (1984). Coronary heart disease mortality in United States blacks, 1940–1978: Trends and unanswered questions. *Am. Heart J., 108*, 728–732.

Glueck, C. J., Gartside, P., Laskarzewski, P. M., et al. (1984). High-density lipoprotein cholesterol in blacks and whites: Potential ramificatinos for coronary heart disease. *Am. Heart J., 108*, 815–826.

Goldman, L. (1990). Cost effectiveness perspectives in coronary heart disease. *Am. Heart J., 119*, 733–740.

Greenberg, M. A., Wiggins, C. L., Kutvist, D. M., & Samet, J. M. (1987). Cigarette use among Hispanic and non-Hispanic white school children in Albuquerque, New Mexico. *Am. J. Public Health, 77*, 621–622.

Grundy, S. (1986). Cholesterol and coronary heart disease: A new era. *JAMA, 256*, 2849.

Johnson, J. L., Heineman, E. F., Heiss, G., et al. (1986). Cardiovascular disease risk factors and mortality among black and white women aged 40–64 years. *Am. J. Epidemiol., 123*, 209–220.

Kannel, W. B. (1981). Update on the role of cigarette smoking in coronary artery disease. *Am. Heart J., 101*, 319–328.

Kwiterovich, P. O., Jr. (1989). Pediatric implications of heterozygous familial hypercholesterolemia. *Arteriosclerosis, 9*(Suppl. I), 111–120.

Lauer R. M., Lee, J., & Clarke, W. R. (1988). Factors affecting the relationship between childhood and adult cholesterol levels: The Muscatine Study. *Pediatrics, 82*, 309–318.

Levy, D., Wilson, P. W., Anderson, K. M., & Castelli, W. P. (1990). Stratifying the patient at risk from coronary disease: New insights from The Framingham Heart Study. *Am. Heart J., 119*, 712–717.

Lifshitz, F., & Moses, N. (1989). Growth failure: A complication of treatment of hypercholesterolemia. *Am J Dis Child, 143*, 537–542.

Lipid Research Clinics Program. (1984). The lipid research clinics coronary trial results: II. The relationship of reduction in incidence of coronary heart disease to cholesterol lowering. *JAMA, 251*, 365–374.

Mead, M. (1943). The problem of changing food habits (Bulletin of the National Research Council No. 108). Washington, DC: Food and Nutrition Board, National Academy of Science.

Miller, S. K., & Slap, G. B. (1989). Adolescent smoking: A review of prevalence and prevention. *J Adol Health Care, 10*, 129–135.

MMWR—Morbidity and Mortality Weekly Report. (1986). Cigarette smoking in the United States. *36*, 581–585.

Moore, T. J. (1989, September). The cholesterol myth. *Atlantic Monthly*, pp. 37–70.

Nicklas, T. A., Frank, G. C., Webbe, L. S., et al. (1987). Racial contrasts in hemoglobin levels and dietary patterns related to hematopoiesis in children: The Bogalusa Heart Study. *Am. J. Public Health, 77*, 1320–1323.

Prineas, R. J., & Gillum, R. (1985). U.S. epidemiology of hypertension in blacks. In D. W. Hall, E. Saunders, & N. B. Shulman (Eds.), *Hypertension in blacks*. Chicago: Yearbook.

Ragland, D. R., & Brand, R. J. (1988). Coronary heart disease mortality in the Western Collaborative Group Study: Follow-up experience of 22 years. *Am. J. Epidemiol., 127*, 462–475.

Schachter, J., Kuller, L. H., & Perfetti, C. (1984). Blood pressure during the first five years of life: Relation to ethnic group (black or white) and to parental hypertension. *Am. J. Epidemiol., 119*, 541–533.

Sempos, C., Cooper, R., Kovar, M. G., & McMillan, M. (1988). Divergence of the recent trends in coronary mortality for the four major race-sex groups in the United States. *Am J Public Health, 78*, 1422–1427.

Stamler, J., Wentworth, D., & Neaton, J. D. (1986). Is the relationship between serum cholesterol and risk from premature death from coronary heart disease continuous or graded? *JAMA, 256*, 2823–2824.

Stavig, G. R., Igra, A., & Leonard, A. R. (1984). Hypertension among Asians and Pacific Islanders in California. *Am.J. Epidemiol., 119*, 677–691.

Tuckson, R. V. (1989). Race, sex, economics and tobacco advertising. *J Nat Med Assoc, 81*, 1119–1124.

Vital Statistics of the United States, 1980 and 1985. (1988). *Mortality* (Vol. 2). Hyattsville, MD: U.S. Department of Health and Human Services, Public Health Service, National Center for Health Statistics.

Wadowski, S. J., Karp, R. J., Bachmann, R., & Senft, C. (1991, April 29). Family history of coronary heart disease and cholesterol screening in a disadvantaged inner-city population. American Pediatric Society/Society for Pediatric Research, New Orleans.

Wallack, L., & Winkleby, M. (1987). Primary prevention: A new look at basic concepts. *Soc. Sci. Med., 25*, 923–930.

Winkleby, M. A., Ragland, D. R., & Syme, S. L. (1988). Heightened risk of hypertension among black males: The masking effects of covariables. *Am J Epidemiol, 128*, 1075–1083.

Winkleby, M. A., Fortmann, S. P., & Barrett, D. C. (1990). Social class disparities in risk factors for disease: Eight-year prevalence patterns by level of education. *Preventive Medicine, 19*, 1–12.

15

Gastroenteritis

Simon Rabinowitz, MD, PhD

Throughout the world, gastroenteritis remains the largest killer of infant children, accounting for 5 to 10 million deaths a year according to the World Health Organization. Almost all of this mortality occurs in the developing world where malnutrition and malabsorption form a vicious cycle that is fueled by acute diarrheal disease. In the United States, the influx of poor immigrants, plus the growing number of impoverished Americans and the increased use of day care centers threaten to make this problem of great concern here. Already, gastroenteritis accounts for 10% of pediatric emergency department visits and a similar number of admissions. Therefore, all pediatric health care workers must have a basic understanding of the pathophysiology of gastroenteritis and the crucial importance of oral rehydration solution to minimize morbidity and mortality.

As the name implies, gastroenteritis is an inflammation involving the stomach and intestines. The overwhelming majority of these episodes are acute infections in children with intact gastrointestinal tracts and no underlying immunological deficits that would impede rapid resolution. However, certain children have abnormalities in either their digestive system or defense barriers that predispose them to more frequent infections with more devastating sequelae. In addition, there are certain noninfectious etiologies for gastroenteritis that need to be considered.

To appreciate the morbidity of gastroenteritis fully, an understanding of its inevitable sequela, malabsorption, is required. Any inflammatory reaction in the gastrointestinal tract, regardless of its etiology, disrupts the normal digestion and absorption of nutrients. It is this disruption that accounts for the consequences of gastroenteritis. In the developing world, where the natural level of reserve is lower, any significant impairment in the supply of nutrients to rapidly growing children may have repercussions. Ironically, it is deficits in the proper absorption of the most elemental and easily absorbable nutrients, sodium and water, that cause the most significant problems. As anyone experienced in primary care pediatrics quickly learns, the combination of diarrhea and dehydration is commonly encountered. The nature of this text, however, does not allow a full discussion of these issues. Suggested readings include Sleisenger and Brandborg (1977), Ulshen (1988), and a Clinicopathologic Exercise from the Massachusetts General Hospital devoted to this topic (1985). The major concern of this chapter is the appropriate use of oral rehydration solutions. Some comments are also appropriate for a recent phenomenon, diarrheal disease in urban day care centers.

GASTROENTERITIS IN DAY CARE CENTERS

Children enrolled in day care centers or any other arrangements that involve multiple children in a given location have an increased incidence of acute diarrheal illness. The problem is greatest among infants and toddlers with fecal incontinence, because the principal mode of transmission is the fecal oral route. Risk of diarrhea seems to be inversely proportional to hand-washing practices especially after diaper changes, and before and after food preparation and consumption. However, direct child-to-child transmission is also an important consideration among toddlers. At present, strict adherence to hygiene is the best available method to minimize gastroenteritis in the day care setting.

A recent report by the Centers for Disease Control found that between 1973 and 1983 there were 500 diarrhea deaths among children less than 4 years of age in the United States. Almost one half occur before 3 months of age and three quarters before 6 months. In every state, black infants are 4 times more likely to die from this condition than white infants. The highest mortality occurs in the Southeast and the winter months when rotavirus is probably most responsible. An in-depth review of data from Mississippi disclosed that death was most common for infants of young (under age 17) unmarried mothers who had not finished high school and had not sought adequate prenatal care (Ho et al., 1988). The single most important factor to prevent unnecessary hospitalization, morbidity, and mortality in the Third World and throughout the United States is the prompt use of oral rehydration therapy.

CLINICIAN'S RESPONSE TO GASTROENTERITIS

The immediate dangers to infants with diarrhea are the consequences of dehydration and electrolyte imbalance. Thus, the first goal is rapid rehydration with an appropriate fluid. In many impoverished areas of the United States as well as most of the developing countries, economic realities dictate the oral administration of such a solution. Indeed after several decades of research and development of oral rehydration solutions, based mainly on children living in impoverished environments, there are still many "private" pediatricians in the United States who rely on parenteral hydration for their patients with acute enteritis. Historically, rice water, barley water, dilute teas, and other home remedies were used for rehydration with limited success. Studies done at the turn of the century and shortly afterward demonstrated the fecal concentration of sodium during diarrheal disease. Subsequently, in the 1950s and 1960s the importance of potassium as well as the wide variation of potassium excretion was appreciated. This led to the first preparation of oral rehydration solutions to treat children with diarrheal diseases.

There are several factors that must be considered in the proper use of oral rehydration.

1. *Degree of dehydration and illness in the individual patient.* Any patient who is suffering from shock, lethargy, and persistent emesis in the emergency department is not a candidate for outpatient care. In virtually all of these situations an initial phase of rapid parenteral hydration is required.
2. *Age of the child.* Younger infants, and especially prematures, have a higher proportion of their body mass as water and have a higher ratio of surface area to body mass than at any other time in their lives.
3. *Nutritional status of the child.* The morbidity and mortality of gastroenteritis is closely related to the degree of wasting and stunting of the child. Martorell (1985) notes that children with reductions in either weight for age (stunting) or weight for length (wasting) are at increased risk for death from infectious illnesses of all types and from gastroenteritis. Children with both wasting and stunting are at the highest risk.

TABLE 15.1 Contents Oral Electrolyte Solutions (per Liter)

	Sodium	Potassium	Other	Cl	Base	Glu
Oral Electrolyte Maintenance Solutions:						
Lytren	30	25	8	25	45	70
Pedialyte	45	20	—	35	30	25
Oral Electrolyte Rehydration Solutions:						
Pedialyte RS	75	20	—	65	30	25
WHO Solution	90	20	—	80	30	20

4. *Etiological agent of gastroenteritis.* The dehydration from a toxigenic bacteria that produces a secretory (high sodium, high potassium) diarrhea needs to be distinguished from the dehydration that results from a rotavirus that may also cause carbohydrate malabsorption.
5. *"Dichotomy" over initial therapeutic fluids versus maintenance fluids.* The aim of some researchers in this field is to devise a single all-purpose rehydration solution. Because of the variations listed earlier this is probably an unrealistic goal. The solutions most commonly used in the United States include Pedialyte and Lytren. These are compared with the World Health Organization recommended formulation in Table 15.1.

Optimally, the malnourished child who is subjected to multiple episodes of these diarrheal illness in the first year of life, is quickly reintroduced to formula after rapid treatment of acute dehydration. The rehydration solution is then supplemented to the normal diet to replace excessive fecal losses in a 1:1 ratio. After rehydration has been achieved a diluted form of the infant's regular formula should be offered for 24 to 72 hours after which time full-strength feedings should be restarted. Although the practice of withholding lactose-containing formulas because of lactose intolerance has become so widespread that the soya protein formulas (lactose free) now account for approximately one third of the formula market in the United States, this is largely unnecessary.

In most infants, a single episode of gastroenteritis will not have any lasting effect. For the infant who is raised in an environment that predisposes to multiple acute infections, including diarrheal illnesses, prompt recognition and institution of oral rehydration therapy is the first step in minimizing morbidity. The second and equally essential component is the reinstitution of energy-containing nutrition. The infant who has several periods of extended undernutrition as a consequence of multiple gastrointestinal infections will have a difficult time maintaining adequate growth and development.

SUMMARY

In summary, health care practitioners should recognize the dangers of diarrheal disease and instruct parents in the rapid and short-term use of standard oral rehydration solutions for affected infants. This will cover most clinical situations.

REFERENCES

Bartlett, A. V., Moore, M., Gary, G. W., et al. (1985). Diarrheal illness among infants and toddlers in day care: I. Epidemiology and pathogens. *Journal of Pediatrics, 106*, 495–502.

Ho, M.-S., Glass, R. I., Pinsky, P. F., et al. (1988). Diarrheal deaths in American children: Are they preventable? *JAMA, 260*, 3281–3285.

Martorell, R. (1985). Child growth retardation: A discussion of its causes and its relationship to health. In K. Blaxter & J. C. Waterlow (Eds.), *Nutritional adaptation in man* (pp. 13–30). London: John Libbey.

Sleisenger, M. H., & Brandborg, L. (1977). *Major problems in internal medicine. Malabsorption*: Vol. 13. Philadelphia: Saunders.

Ulshen, M. H. (1988). Refeeding during recovery from acute diarrhea. *Journal of Pediatrics, 112*, 239–240.

(1985). Weekly clinicopathological exercises. *313, NEJM*, 805–815.

16

Growth and Nutrition During Adolescent Pregnancy

Theresa O. Scholl, PhD, MPH,
Mary L. Hediger, PhD,
Peter Vasilenko III, PhD,
Mary F. Healy, RD

In this chapter we consider the effect of prenatal nutrition in the pregnant adolescent on the health of the fetus, the newborn, and the mother herself after delivery. The United States has one of the highest rates of pregnancy and childbearing in young women under the age of 20 of any Western industrialized nation (National Center for Health Statistics, 1989). Currently, in Camden, New Jersey, adolescents make up 17% of all pregnancies.

Low birth weight is a leading cause of infant mortality and child morbidity in the United States. As shown in the Figure 16.1, achieving a birth weight above 2.5 kg, for the most part, is associated with reduced infant mortality. For any group of infants, moving the distribution curve to the right (higher mean birth weight) is associated with better infant survival because there are fewer low-birth-weight infants (Rush, 1980).

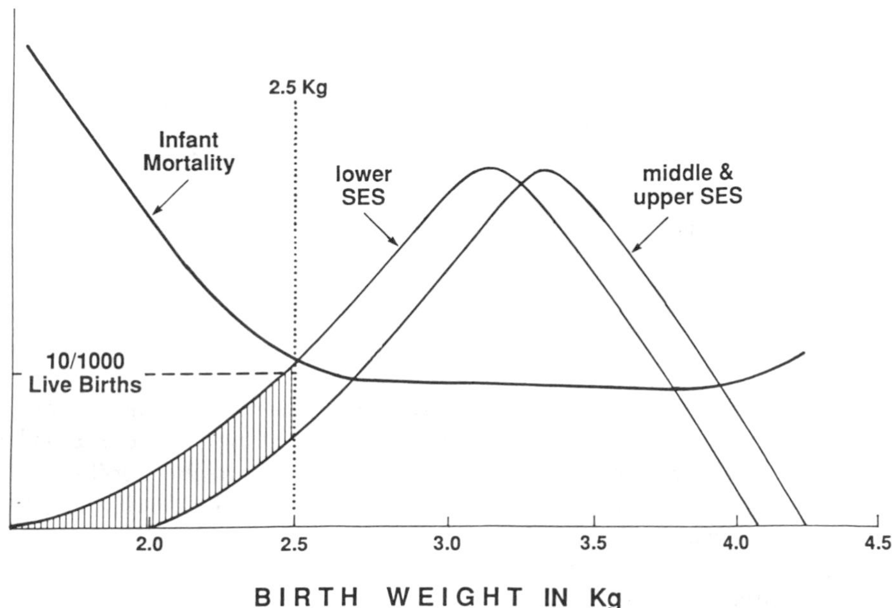

FIGURE 16.1 While the difference in mean birth weight between the highest and lowest socioeconomic status groups may seem small (about 150 grams), this difference is associated with a substantial increase in the number of LBW infants. The darkened area represents the resultant increase in infant mortality.

An increased risk of low birth weight associated with adolescent pregnancy is well known (Committee to Study the Prevention of Low Birthweight, 1985). For the mother, a prior history of bearing a low-birth-weight infant is one of the strongest risk factors for a subsequently similar poor outcome. Risk factors often present in young gravidas of low socioeconomic status include smoking, drinking, and drug use during pregnancy; being an ethnic minority; and inadequate prenatal care in addition to factors indicative of poor nutritional status (e.g., anemia, low prepregnant weight, and inadequate gestational gains). To this list, we add an additional nutritional factor—continued maternal growth during adolescent pregnancy (Scholl, Hediger, Ances, & Cronk, 1988; Scholl, Hediger, & Ances, 1990).

MATERNAL GROWTH DURING PREGNANCY

A growth spurt occurs during adolescence, involving all skeletal and muscular dimensions, and almost every other system and organ of the

TABLE 16.1 Variables to Consider in Assessing Health and Nutritional Status in Adolescents

Variable	Range
Age at onset of adolescence	10 to 14 years
Increment following:	
peak height velocity	10.8 to 22.3 cm
menarche	7.11 to 10.6 cm
Time after menarche that growth continues	3.8 to 6.7 years

body, except the brain and head (Tanner, 1972). During adolescence, weight is gained at about the same rate as in infancy and childhood; linear growth has a considerably lower velocity (Marschall & Tanner, 1989). As shown in Table 16.1, measures of adolescent growth and maturity vary greatly.

Linear growth is the preferred marker of continuing development since, unlike weight, it cannot occur after growth ceases (Frisancho, 1985). At age 17, approximately 50% of young white women from the Fels Longitudinal Study achieved mature stature while the remainder continued linear growth through age 20 or 21 (Roche & Davilla, 1972).

As a result of growth, adolescent nutritional requirements exceed those of mature women. However, given the normal variation in timing and rate of growth, adolescent nutritional requirements probably depend more on whether growth is continuing or has ceased than on chronological age (Dwyer, 1981). Thus, when a teenager is pregnant, the availability of nutrients to the fetus or the mother will depend, in part, on whether or not a young mother continues to grow while she is pregnant (Jacobson, 1983). Menarche usually is subsequent to the peak of the height spurt and occurs at a time when height velocity is decreasing (Tanner, 1972). A period of subfertility usually follows so that pregnancy should be relatively uncommon in rapidly growing girls (Beal, 1981). However, pregnant adolescents have an increased likelihood of being early maturers (Hoff et al., 1989). Thus, they may be expected to show greater amounts of postmenarcheal growth (Tanner, 1972), but a shorter interval of anovulatory cycles than later maturing adolescents (Apter & Viho, 1985).

It has been suggested that maternal growth is an underlying cause of the increased rate of complications and poor outcomes that characterize adolescent pregnancy (Frisancho et al., 1985). Adolescents with early age at menarche have an increased risk of low-birth-weight and

SGA births associated with their own continued growth (Scholl, Hediger, Vasilenko, et al., 1989). Conversely, adolescents of low gynecological age, defined as a conception within two completed years of menarche *without regard to age at menarche,* have an increased risk of preterm birth (Scholl, Hediger, Salmon, et al., 1989). This view is in contrast to a widely held view that maternal growth during pregnancy is of little potential consequence for mother or fetus (Forbes, 1981). Until recently, an accepted teaching has been that the small amount of linear growth observed in U.S. gravidas was unlikely to be clinically important, to threaten maternal nutritional status, or to compromise fetal growth. As we will show, this belief reflects the inappropriate measuring methods used by the investigators.

NEW TECHNIQUE TO ASSESS GROWTH—KNEE HEIGHT MEASUREMENT

Our own prospective and ongoing study of growth during adolescent pregnancy indicates the methods used to detect maternal growth in past studies are insensitive, given special conditions that exist during pregnancy (Scholl, Hediger, & Ances, 1990). Maternal growth, measured using change in knee height, with the Knee Height Measuring Devise (KHMD) (Cronk et al., 1989) occurs in about 50% of adolescent primigravidas and multigravidas with a first pregnancy at 12 to 15 years. Growth of young pregnant women is not clinically apparent; it is masked by the tendency of gravidas of all ages to shrink slightly, but significantly, in stature during the course of pregnancy. Thus, the reliance on serial measurements of stature has seriously underestimated the number of young gravidas who are growing and the amount of maternal growth that occurs during pregnancy.

MATERNAL NUTRITIONAL STATUS DURING ADOLESCENT PREGNANCY

Adolescents may be more dependent on gestational gains than mature controls (Frisancho et al., 1985). Early weight gain adequacy may be a particular problem among adolescent gravidas because of their tendencies to poor prepregnant nutritional status, nutritionally poor diets during pregnancy, and body image concerns, but it is not known if irregular patterns of weight gain during adolescent pregnancy are associated with birth weight and length of gestation. We studied weight gain during pregnancy and pregnancy outcome in a cohort of 1,790 low-income teenage gravidas who entered prenatal care before 24 weeks' gestation (Hediger, Scholl, Belsky, Ances, & Salmon et al., 1989). We found that 17.0% of the cohort had inadequate weight gain early in gestation and that early inadequate gains alone were associated with a twofold increase in risk of having a SGA infant. Late inadequate gains were associated significantly with preterm delivery as well as SGA babies, even if the total gain was adequate for gestation. Thus, pregnant teenagers who purposefully or inadvertently limit their weight gain early in pregnancy, so that it falls below recommended standards for adults, are at increased risk of having a growth-retarded infant.

DIET DURING ADOLESCENT PREGNANCY

Inadequate weight gain during pregnancy is thus an important risk factor for low birth weight, but the contribution of diet to inadequate weight gain for gestation is uncertain. The effects of diet on inadequate weight gain for gestation were studied in a random sample of 370 Camden teenagers, who had a single dietary 24-hour recall taken at entry to prenatal care (averaging 17 weeks' gestation). The course of their pregnancies was followed through delivery. Inadequate weight gain was defined using clinical standards that correspond to a gain of less than 2.9 kg at 20 weeks' gestation or approximated 400 g/week or less thereafter until delivery (Scholl, Hediger, Koo et al., 1988). We found, after adjusting for potential confounding variables, that teenagers with inadequate weight gain for gestation had consumed approximately 300 calories less than teenagers with adequate weight gain ($p < .05$) (Scholl et al., 1990). Significant deficits were found in protein and carbohydrate intake associated with inadequate weight gain, also. In a second study involving mature women and teenagers, significant diminished intake of calories (– 167), protein (– 6.5 g), fat (– 8.1 g), and zinc (– 1.0 mg), and borderline differences in iron (– 2.3 mg) and folacin (– 37.4 μg) was present in teen gravidas with poor weight gain. Control for calories resulted in virtually identical point estimates between those with adequate and inadequate gain, suggesting that weight gain is primarily energy driven.

NUTRIENT INTAKE AND PREGNANCY OUTCOME

In laboratory animals, nutrient deficiencies, induced by controlled feeding experiments, are clearly related to an increased rate of retarded growth and congenital defects in the fetus, whereas human studies are inconsistent (Leiberman et al., 1987). One nutrient deficiency (zinc) is associated with retarded postnatal growth and development (King et al., 1987). Administration of iron may also be associated with reduced maternal zinc during pregnancy, perhaps inducing iatrogenic zinc deficiency (Dawson et al., 1989). Complicating the issue is the fact that serum or plasma zinc is more of a screening than a diagnostic test for poor zinc status, but there is no preferred indicator that is available (Solomons, 1988).

Apart from anemia the functional consequences of low stores of iron and folate are unknown, although poor maternal folate status has been associated with neural tube defects during pregnancy (Medical Research Council, 1991). Because of methodological problems in analyzing the folate content of food, intake may be inadequate to assess folate status (Suhar et al., 1989). Studies examining pregnancy outcome associated with anemia have indicated increased risks of preterm birth, SGA, and low birth weight with both low and high maternal hemoglobin and hematocrit (Leiberman et al., 1987), as well as with serum ferritin and plasma folate (Kramer, 1987). These findings may be attributable, in part, to failure to control for gestation and resulting hematological changes.

Thus, low levels of nutrients may serve as a marker for other risk factors associated with poor outcome or may themselves be confounded by failure to control for gestation or other maternal characteristics. In other cases, a deficiency of one or more micronutrients may be induced by inadequate diet, failure to replete maternal nutrient stores following pregnancy, supplementation with another nutrient, or increased nutrient requirements, say, for maternal growth and for pregnancy.

COMPETITION FOR NUTRIENTS BETWEEN MOTHER AND FETUS

We have observed a weak association between maternal growth and infant birth weight in primigravidas ages 12 to 15, but a substantial decrement (– 100 g in birth weight/millimeter increase in knee height) in the growing multiparous adolescent, even after control for confounding variables (Scholl et al., 1990). The absolute difference in birth weight amounted to nearly 300 g. Data from *primigravidas* were therefore consistent with the observation that U.S. adolescents are able to support a pregnancy, even in the face of growth (Sukanich et al., 1986). But the data for *multigravidas* (increased risk of low birth weight, preterm delivery, and infant mortality) suggest otherwise. As hypothesized by Naeye (1981) and Rosso (1981) there may be a competition for nutrients between a still-growing mother and her fetus, which may involve reduced uteroplacental blood flow to conserve maternal nutrient stores.

Lack of availability of nutrients may upset the balance between mother and fetus during pregnancy, and engender a competition for nutrients as the maternal body attempts to maintain its stores. Pregnant adolescents have been hypothesized to have an increased likelihood of competing with their fetuses for essential nutrients because of continuing growth (Frisancho et al., 1985). It has been suggested that placental function is contingent on maternal nutritional status. That is, when nutrients are abundant the placenta acts as a fetal organ and transmits freely to the fetus. When nutrient status is compromised, the placenta uses nutrients for its own metabolism at the expense of the fetus (Picone et al., 1982).

After the first delivery many women make a physiological transition that allows them in subsequent pregnancies to nourish the developing fetus better (Hytten & Chamberlain, 1980). As noted earlier, in mature women, multiparity usually is associated with a decreased risk of low birth weight and an increase in birth weight. This response does not occur for the multiparous adolescent where birth weight either decreases or fails to improve with parity (Scholl et al., 1988). Although studies of this phenomenon are limited, publications based on National Center for Health Statistics data (1980) or that included a stratum of young gravidas have noted the phenomenon (McCormack et al., 1984).

Parity and young maternal age are also associated with short spacing between successive pregnancies, increasing the likelihood of low birth weight, SGA births, and neonatal mortality. Failure to recover from the preceding pregnancy and to replete nutritional stores may occur when pregnancies are closely spaced, as they are in multiparous women under the age of 20 (Kramer, 1987). This problem would seem to be made more acute if coupled with continued maternal growth.

SUMMARY

Poor nutrition is strongly correlated with the social and economic milieu that gives rise to adolescent pregnancy. Our research, controlling for many of the suboptimal circumstances in which many young mothers were raised, suggests that many of the adverse outcomes associated with an early pregnancy have a nutritional component. The anabolic needs of mother and fetus may not be met by dietary intakes and, in the case of still-growing multiparous adolescents, nutritional stores may be depleted by rapid repeat child-bearing.

Although evidence is still incomplete, adolescents who are pregnant do appear to be more sensitive to the effects of nutrition than mature women. Secondary prevention involving the remediation of inadequate maternal nutritional status is important, particularly early in pregnancy, to prevent low birth weight and SGA. However, we should always be cognizant of the importance of primary prevention of pregnancy in teenagers many of whom are adolescent and therefore still developing in body as well as in mind.

Case Study from Kings County Hospital
Rene Murray-Bachmann, MS, RD

Tracy Q. is a 14-year-old teen mother who lives with her son, Ibn, her mother, Sarah, and her 13-year-old brother, Randy. The family practices a form of Islam. Both Tracy and her mother wear a full khiddar, a garb that allows only the eyes and bridge of the nose to be exposed. This dress made it difficult to detect Tracy's pregnancy until nearly 5 months had passed.

Sarah attempted to obtain prenatal care for Tracy at a Department of Health clinic, but they were too late in the pregnancy for enrollment in the community health center. Tracy received no care until 34 weeks' gestation when her "water broke," and she was brought by the emergency medical service to Kings County Hospital. She delivered a vigorous infant shortly after arrival. Ibn weighed 1,920 g at birth, which was appropriate for the gestational age.

Ibn did not gain weight and was kept in the neonatal intensive care unit, then the intermediate care unit, until he weighed 2,500 g, which took 4 weeks. Though it was stated on the hospital record that Tracy was 15 years old and planned to breast- and bottle-feed, at no time during the admission was she seen by the ward dietitian. "Not necessary" was checked off under diet instructions in her discharge summary. At his first visit to the Pediatric Resource Center (PRC), at 8 weeks of age (4 weeks after discharge), Ibn weighed approximately the same as at discharge. Our evaluation involved several members of the health care team, each of whom received somewhat different information by the mother. The pediatric resident who saw the child initially was given a glowing history of a child with a vigorous appetite. When the health educator spoke with the mother she found that Tracy was diluting the iron-fortified formula with an extra can or two of water, lowering the calorie concentration from 20 to 15, or 10 calories per ounce. The dietitian (myself) found that for Tracy, breast-feeding meant leaving Ibn on one breast for a few minutes and then changing to the other, thus limiting caloric intake. I also found that the family was polygamous.

The nurses drew Sarah into the discussion to make sure that she took responsibility for seeing that Ibn was fed. The staff pediatrician reviewed the measurement, ordered some baseline laboratory tests and, with the dietitian, developed a treatment plan. No social worker was available to see the family at that time.

Small feedings at frequent intervals were encouraged. Tracy was encouraged to empty her breasts completely several times a day, but the main feeding was iron-fortified infant formula. The grandmother, Sarah, was instructed to mix one can of concentrate with one can of water and to add two teaspoonfuls of olive oil to the large container to raise the caloric content of the formula. Multivitamin drops with iron were given. The important concern was whether the baby would gain the 30 g a day, suggestive of adequate feeding. All instructions were written down and reviewed with Sarah and Tracy, both of whom understood our concern. They were instructed to return in 48 hours for a weight check. In the late afternoon, Ibn, Tracy, and Sarah arrived, to the relief of the staff involved. The social workers were there and raised some new concerns. If this was a polygamous family, why were the other wives not involved in the care of the infant? Polygamous families generally share responsibilities. Why was the care of Ibn so ineffective?

And why were they late? Sarah told us with great irritation that Tracy had forgotten to mention an important test scheduled for the morning. Though never threatened, Sarah was streetwise and knew the consequence of not showing up for the appointment was a child-neglect report. We weighed Ibn. He had gained 120 g in 2 days. Everyone cheered. We were all very positive and reassuring with the family.

At this time, Sarah's husband, Hassan, arrived in the clinic. He berated his wife and daughter. "You did not tell me where you were, and you came to Kings County Hospital." He told me angrily that he was the father of 12 children and knew perfectly well how to take care of them himself.

I was as calm as I could be, given the nature of this "conversation." I explained that Ibn had failure to thrive and required extra special attention that we at the PRC were doing our best to provide. We spoke of Tracy's youth and her need for support. Mr. Q. protested loudly that teen pregnancy was the will of Allah. He was also adamant that the baby and the mother be seen by a woman physician only. Because these comments do not derive from normative Islam, I was concerned that the poor nutrition might reflect a form of cult behavior. But the request of the family was honored. Care of Ibn was transferred to a woman physician.

The social workers suggested that the other wives come to the next appointment, and, 5 days later, another wife, Sondra, came to the PRC with the family. In chapter 20, Dr. Bradley describes the role of the "pivotal person" in a family who makes important decisions. The principal wife, Sondra, was that person. Ibn showed an additional 300-g gain to 2,950 g. Tracy smiled for the first time, and jumped up and down with excitement.

DIETS FOR TRACY

1. Before delivery—a diet for the pregnant adolescent
   2200 calories—base line requirement
   300 calories—usual need for pregnant adults
   350 calories—supplement during second and third trimester for adolescents
   2800 calories—a minimal total caloric intake
2. After delivery—a diet for the breast-feeding adolescent

As Scholl and her colleagues have shown, it is essential to maintain sufficient caloric intake for both lactation and her own growth.

2200 calories—base line requirement
500 calories—for lactation
300 calories—to maintain her own growth

Extensive supplementation of vitamins and minerals are essential. An important consideration is calcium loss during the lactation of a teen mother (Chan et al., 1987). Providing the needed foods depends a great deal on the culture of the family. The Q. family observes biblical dietary laws that must be respected (see chapter 12). They were not, however, food cultists. Liquids are important to allow proper let-down and refilling. If possible 8 oz of milk should be served with each of the three main meals. If there is lactose intolerance, use of low-lactose dairy products (yogurt and naturally aged cheeses) are suggested or, alternatively, commercially produced lactase may be recommended with lactose-containing dairy products.

REFERENCES

Apter, D., & Vihko, R. (1985). Premenarcheal endocrine changes in relation to age at menarche. *Clin Endocrinol, 22*, 753–760.

Beal, V. A. (1981). Assessment of nutritional status in pregnancy. *Am J Clin Nutr, 34*(Suppl.), 691–696.

Chan, G. M., McMurray, M., Westouer, K., et al. (1987). Effects of dietary calcium intake upon the calcium and bone mineral status of lactating adolescents and adults. *Am J Clin Nutrition, 46*, 319–323.

CSPLB—Committee to Study the Prevention of Low Birthweight. (1985). *Preventing low birthweight.* Washington, DC: National Academy Press.

Cronk, C. E., Stallings, V. A., Spender, Q. W., Ross, J. L., & Widdoes, H. D. (1989). Measurement of short term growth with a new knee height measuring device (KHMD). *Am J Hum Biol, 1*, 421–428.

Dawson, E. B., Albers, J., & McGanity, W. J. (1989). Serum zinc changes due to iron supplementation in teen-age pregnancy. *Am J Clin Nutr, 50*, 848–852.

Dwyer, J. (1981). Nutritional requirements of adolescence. *Nutrition Review, 39*, 56–72.

Forbes, G. B. (1981). Pregnancy in the teenager: Biologic aspects. In *Pregnancy and childbearing during adolescence: Birth defects* (Original Articles Series, March of Dimes Birth Defects Foundation, Vol. 17, pp. 85–90). New York: Liss.

Frisancho, A. R., Matos, J., Leonard, W. R., & Yaroch, L. A. (1985). Developmental and nutritional determinants of pregnancy outcome among teenagers. *Am J Phys Anthrop, 66*, 247–261.

Hediger, M. L., Scholl, T. O., Belsky, D. H., Ances, I. G., & Salmon, R. W. (1989). Patterns of weight gain in adolescent pregnancy: effects on birth weight and preterm delivery. *Obstet Gynecol, 74*, 6–12.

Hoff, C., Wertelecki, W., Zansky, S., et al. (1985). Earlier maturation of pregnant black and white adolescents. *Am J Dis Child, 139*, 981–986.

Hytten, F., & Chamberlain, G. (1980). *Clinical physiology in obstetrics.* London: Blackwell Scientific.

Jacobson, M. S., & Heald, F. P. (1983). Nutritional risks of adolescent pregnancy and their management. E. R. McAnarney (Ed.), *Premature adolescent pregnancy and parenthood* (pp. 119–135). New York: Grune & Stratton.

King, J. C., Bronstein, M. N., Fitch, W., et al. (1987). Nutrient utilization during pregnancy. *Wld. Rev. Nutr. Diet, 52*, 71–142.

Kramer, M. F. (1987). Determinants of low birth weight: Methodological assessment and meta-analysis. *Bulletin WHO, 65*, 663–737.

Lieberman, E., Ryan, K. J., Monson, R. R., et al. (1987). Medical and socioeconomic characteristics accounting for racial differences in rates of premature births. *New England Journal of Medicine, 317*, 743–748.

Marshall, W. A., & Tanner, J. M. (1969). Variations in patterns of pubertal changes in girls. *Arch Dis Child, 44*, 291–303.

McCormick, M., Shapiro, S., & Starfield, B. (1984). High-risk young mothers: Infant mortality and morbidity in four areas in the United States, 1973–1978. *Am J Public Health, 74*, 18–21.

Medical Research Council. (1991). Prevention of neural tube defects: Results of the Medical Research Council Vitamin Study. *Lancet, 338*, 131–137.

Naeye, R. L. (1981). Teenaged and pre-teenaged pregnancies: Consequences of the fetal-maternal competition for nutrients. *Pediatrics, 67*, 146–150.

National Center for Health Statistics. (1980). Factors associated with low birthweight: United States, 1976. (Vital and Health Statistics, Series 21, No. 37). (DHHS Publication No. [PHS] 80–1915). Hyattsville, MD: Public Health Service.

National Center for Health Statistics. (1989). Advance report of final maternity statistics, 1987. *Monthly Vital Statistics Report, 38*, 1–48.

Picone, T. A., Allen, L. H., Olsen, P., et al. (1982). Pregnancy outcome in North American women: II. Effects of diet, cigarette smoking, stress and weight gain on placentas and on neonatal physical and behavioral characteristics. *Am J Clin Nutr, 36*, 1214–1224.

Roche, A. R., & Davila, G. H. (1972). Late adolescent growth in stature. *Pediatrics, 50*, 874–880.

Rosso, P. (1981). Nutrition and maternal-fetal exchange. *Am J Clin Nutr, 34*(Suppl.), 744–755.

Rush, D. E., Stein, Z., Susser., M., et al. (1980). *Diet in pregnancy: A randomized controlled trial of nutritional supplements* (Birth Defects Original Article Series, Vol. 16). New York: Liss.

Scholl, T. O., Hediger, M. L., & Ances, I. G. (1990). Maternal growth during pregnancy and decreased infant birth weight. *Am J Clin Nutr, 51*, 790–793.

Scholl, T. O., Hediger, M. L., Ances, I. G., & Cronk, C. E. (1988). Growth during early teenage pregnancies. *Lancet, 1:*, 701–702 and *2*, 738.

Scholl, T. O., Hediger, M., Koo, C. S., et al. (1991). Maternal weight gain, diet and infant birth weight: Correlations during adolescent pregnancy. *J Clin Epidemiology, 44*, 423–428.

Scholl, T. O., Hediger, M. L., Salmon, R. W., et al. (1989). The influence of prepregnant body mass and weight gain for gestation on spontaneous preterm delivery and duration of gestation during adolescent pregnancy. *Am J Human Biology, 1*, 657–664.

Scholl, T. O., Hediger, M. L., Vasilenko, P., Ances, I. G., Smith, W., & Salmon, R. W. (1989). Effects of early maturation on fetal growth. *Ann Hum Biol, 16*, 335–345.

Solomons, N. (1989). Zinc and copper. In M. E. Shils, & V. Young (Eds.), *Modern nutrition in health and disease.* (6th ed., pp. 238–262). Philadelphia: Lea & Febiger.

Suhar, A. F., Block, G., & James, L. D. (1989). Folate intake and food sources in the U.S. population. *Am J Clin Nutr, 50*, 508–516.

Sukanich, A. C., Rogers, K. D., & McDonald, H. M. (1986). Physical maturity and outcome of pregnancy in primiparas younger than 16 years of age. *Pediatrics, 78*, 31–36.

Tanner, J. M. (1972). *Growth at adolescence* (2nd ed.). Oxford: Blackwell Scientific.

17

Oral Care for the Disadvantaged Child

Diane L. Markowitz, DMD

Disadvantaged children do not suffer from different kinds of oral disease than do their more well-nourished peers. There is considerable evidence, however, that the poorer general health and social conditions of both the child and family contribute to an increase in the severity of their dental problems (Pinkham, 1988), the most common of which are caries—and later in life—peridontal disease (Sutcliffe et al., 1984).

For the infant, the mouth is the portal through which food, affection, and even information pass. It is also no less a mirror of the total health of an individual than is any other area of the body, yet the oral cavity is rarely perceived as requiring much care in the very young. In fact, it is in early childhood that patterns of nutrition and personal hygiene are developed that influence oral health throughout the individual's lifetime.

Finally, the conditions that contribute to and accompany poverty often place children at greater risk for abuse (Giangrego, 1986), and the mouth is not infrequently the site of injury. For all these reasons, it is essential that all health care workers be able to identify both health and disease in the oral cavity and understand when and to whom to refer patients for specialized care.

DIET AND DENTAL DISEASE

Although much attention has been devoted in the literature to the alterations noted in oral mucous membrane and gingival health when there is malnutrition, these changes in the oral cavity are not uniquely pathognomonic of particular nutritional deficiencies. Common dietary practices and a few of the most frequently seen vitamin and mineral deficiencies are actually responsible for the majority of oral symptoms. Zinc deficiency, as found in the United States, contributes to both a depression in the immune response to disease and a decrease in sensitivity to sweet taste (see chapter 18). Children suffering from malnutrition thus frequently crave sweets and, if provided with them in sufficient quantity, will develop rampant decay (Miller, 1982). Though the natural desire for sweets diminishes with age, susceptibility to the dental effects of continual sugar ingestion remains high throughout adolescence (Desor & Beauchamp, 1987).

The frequency of exposure to sweets is directly correlated with the incidence of caries. *Streptococcus Mutans*, the causative agent of tooth decay, requires a fermentable substrate of dietary sugar for metabolism. The practices of adding sugar or honey to liquids fed through nursing bottles, of allowing the infant to fall asleep with a bottle of milk, juice, or infant formula; or of continuing bottle feeding beyond 15 or 16 months can lead to "nursing bottle syndrome" (Goepford, 1987). The result is decay of the anterior dentition—and eventually, the molars, as well—so extensive that intense pain and infection occur, requiring extraction of affected teeth. Typically, also, oral hygiene is poor, with an accumulation of debris and plaque—*Materia Alba*—encircling the teeth and an edematous gingival margin. At greatest risk are children of single-parent families, seen by caregivers as strong-tempered and having difficulty sleeping (Marino et al., 1989). Of special concern is the high rate of baby bottle tooth decay among Native American children (Broderick et al., 1989).

Failure to treat badly decayed deciduous teeth can lead to alveolar abscess with pain, chronic infection, and even eventual destruction of the succedaneous teeth. Because premature loss of deciduous molars allows the remaining teeth to drift toward the front of the mouth, the child who does not receive restorations or space-maintaining appliances is condemned to a severely crowded permanent dentition. Moreover, orthodontic care may be unavailable to such children, as the Medicaid programs of most states severely restrict reimbursement for orthodontics.

PREVENTION

Virtually all dental decay and periodontal disease are preventable. Other than good oral hygiene and avoidance of sweets, the most effective method of reducing decay have pit and fissure sealants of permanent teeth (Straffon & Dennison, 1988) and the introduction of 1 part per million fluoride into community water supplies. In areas where there is no natural fluoridation, this measure has succeeded in decreasing the decay rate by 17% to 40% (McCann, 1989). As a result, children in fluoridated urban areas do not experience rampant decay unless the teeth are constantly bathed in cariogenic fluids. Rural areas, in which 40% of America's poor live are usually not fluoridated, however, and this fact is reflected in a high rate of decay. Such areas also comprise 80% of the locations underserved by dentists in this country, areas in which there is only one dentist for 5,000 or more individuals in the community (Waldman, 1989). To give these children the advantage that fluoridated water confers, a fluoride supplement can be prescribed, either in pill (to be dissolved under the tongue or chewed) or liquid form with a daily dose of 0.25 mg (to age 2), 0.5 mg (to age 3), and 1.0 mg (older than 3 years of age until all the permanent teeth have erupted) (American Academy of Pediatrics, 1979). In addition, school programs in which children are supervised while they brush, floss, and rinse with a fluoride solution have been found to be very effective in reducing decay (Sutcliffe et al., 1984).

The utility of such programs has been found to be far superior to programs that attempt to influence parental behavior (Feldman, 1988). The placement of dental care facilities in the school or provision of transportation to dental clinics has been very successful in improving the oral health of children not otherwise served.

NEGLECT AND ABUSE

Few states define neglect regarding a child's oral health such that failure to seek care is an actionable offense. Only when care has been demonstrated to be available and the need for treatment is obvious to a lay person can true neglect be said to have occurred (Loochtan et al., 1986). Parents must be advised in the strongest possible terms of the consequences of failure to have dental disease treated and reminded specifically of their responsibilities.

Dental disease is rarely brought to the attention of the dentist in cases of neglect or abuse. Physicians and nurses, who are more likely to see these children regularly, are in a better position to observe decay before it becomes rampant. They are also more likely to note the signs of abuse, even without a complete physical examination, as orofacial trauma is present in approximately 50% of cases of physical abuse (Needleman, 1986). The most common explanation given by caregivers for orofacial trauma is a fall, and, indeed, children do fall and do sustain injury to the teeth and face in a variety of ways that should not engender suspicion in the clinician. The type of trauma, however, should be appropriate to the developmental stage of the child. The clinical signs to be investigated further include

1. *Soft-tissue injuries to more than one plane of the face.* Children normally put their hands out when falling, making serious injury to the face unlikely. Despite this, lacerations to the chin are not uncommon and may be accompanied by a subcondylar fracture that, if untreated, may result in a permanent facila deformity. Signs of such a fracture include pain, trismus, and deviation to the affected side on opening. These children should be referred to a maxillofacial surgeon for treatment.
2. *Multiple bruises or lacerations in various stages of healing.* This includes intraoral scarring in more than one location as well as extraoral bruises that display the clear impression of fingers or thumb, or a gag (Schmitt, 1986).
3. *Traumatic loss (avulsion), intrusion, or lingual depression of previously erupted teeth before the appropriate time for the teeth to be lost.* It is not uncommon for a toddler to sustain a fracture to a maxillary incisor and even a detachment of the labial frenum in the process of learning to walk. The sequelae of such injuries may include root fracture, discoloration of the tooth, and abscess, all requiring treatment by a pediatric dentist or endodontist. An accompanying alveolar fracture with bony mobility, however, is likely to have been caused by a blow of more force than that resulting from an ordinary fall.
4. *Injuries to the soft palate.* Although children do occasionally injure the soft palate by falling while holding a toy or similar object in the mouth, soft palate injury can be a common finding in forcible fellatio (Schmitt, 1986).
5. *Facial fractures.* These are relatively uncommon in children unless they have been assaulted.

ACCESS TO CARE

Despite numerous federally and state-funded programs that provide dental treatment for children, fewer than 25% of those eligible, in many locations, receive care (Waldman, 1988, 1989). Some public programs that do exist include

1. In cooperation with Head Start, the Public Health Service provides dental consultants who arrange and provide care for children enrolled in the Head Start program. Unfortunately, only one in five eligible children is enrolled in Head Start (Beck, 1985).
2. The federal Maternal and Child Health Program provides block grants to states for child health care, but dental care generally does not have a high priority, and, in fact, only 35 states currently have dental directors to request and arrange for the use of such aid.
3. Large metropolitan areas, such as New York City, have a variety of programs available to serve eligible children, but most have had to reduce services periodically because of governmental budget cuts and shortfalls of private donations (see chapter 23) Many children do not receive care because their parents, though poor, are not eligible for aid or simply do not know how to enroll in programs for which they are eligible. In one survey, only 40% of homeless children had Medicaid, and 60% had not sought dental care in the previous year, because they had no money or dental insurance (Miller & Lin, 1988).
4. The Indian Health Service provides treatment for Native American children who are enrolled in Head Start programs, but, again, few of those eligible are enrolled. In addition, the prevalence in this population of conditions requiring extensive treatment, such as nursing bottle syndrome, places a heavy burden on a relatively small group of practitioners (see chapter 19).

The picture that emerges is one of a lack of national commitment to good oral health for all of our children. Inadequate funding and haphazard application of preventive measures combine to create a new generation of adults at increased risk for decay, periodontal disease, and tooth loss. They comprise a conspicuous underclass, handicapped by poor oral health and easily identifiable by their unattractive appearance.

REFERENCES

American Academy of Pediatrics, Committee on Nutrition. (1979). Fluoride supplementation: Revised dosage schedule. *Pediatrics, 63*, 150–152.

Beck, R. W. (1985). An overview of maternal and child health dental activities and the Dental Head Start Program. *J. Public Health Dent., 45*, 232–233.

Broderick, E., Mabry, J., Robertson, D., & Thompson, J. (1989). Baby bottle tooth decay in Native American children in Head Start centers. *Pub Health Rep., 104*, 50–54.

Desor, J. A., & Beauchamp, G. K. (1987). Longitudinal changes in sweet preferences in humans. *Physiol Behav., 39*, 639–641.

Feldman, C. A., et al. (1988). The rural Dental Health Program: Long-term impact of two dental delivery systems on children's oral health. *48*, 201–7.

Giangrego, E. (1986). Child abuse: Recognition and reporting. *Spec. Care Dentist, 6*, 62–67.

Goepferd, S. J. (1987). An infant oral health program: The first 18 months. *Pediatr. Dent., 9*, 8–12.

Loochtan, R. M., et al. (1986). Dental neglect in children: Definition, legal aspects and challenges. *Pediatr Dent, 8*, 101–102.

Marino, R. U., et al. (1989). Nursing bottle caries: Characteristics of children at risk. *Clin. Pediatr., 28*, 129–131.

McCann, D. (1989). Fluoride and oral health: A story of achievements and challenges. *J. Am. Dent. Assoc., 118*, 529–540.

Miller, D. S., & Lin, H. B. (1988). Children in sheltered homeless families: Reported health status and use of health services. *Pediatrics, 81*, 668–673.

Miller, J., Vaughan-Williams, E., Furlong, R., & Harrison, L. (1982). Dental caries and children's weights. *J. Epidem. Commun. Health, 36*, 49–52.

Needleman, H. L. (1986). Orofacial trauma in child abuse: Types, prevalence, management, and the dental profession's involvement. *Pediatr. Dent., 8*, 71–80.

Pinkham, J., et al. (1988). Dentistry and the children of poverty. *J. Dent. Child., 6*, 452–454.

Schmitt, B. D. (1986). Physical abuse: specifics of clinical diagnosis. *Pediatr. Dent., 8*, 83–87.

Straffon, L. H., & Dennison, J. B. (1988). Clinical evaluation comparing sealant and amalgam after 7 years: A final report. *J Am Dent Assoc., 117*, 751–755.

Sutcliffe, P., Raynor, J. A., & Brown, M. (1984). Daily supervised tooth brushing in nursery school. *Br. Dent. J., 157*, 201–204.

Waldman, B. H. (1988). And what of children? *J Dent Child., 55*, 418–421.

Waldman, B. H. (1989). Continuing potential for pediatric dental services in nonurban areas. *J. Dent. Child, 56*, 216–219.

Part III
Prevention and Intervention

Malnutrition is as often a symptom of disadvantage and poverty as it is a consequence. It is best treated by an interdisciplinary team including the physician, nurse(s), nutritionist, social worker, and home health worker. Coordination with community agencies is also essential, but Bureaus of Child Welfare are often available only at a point that is very late in the development of the cycle of poverty. Other groups, such as food programs, schools, day-care centers, libraries, parenting groups, and private social and religious groups, can prevent the cycle of poverty from ever occurring.

There are barriers to health care and to good health for the poor. In the United States, there is a lack of both adequate health insurance and adequate public facilities. Without health insurance, the disadvantaged cannot use the private system for health care. For the most disadvantaged children, health care services required are found in the under-funded public sector. Without adequate resources, much of the preventive efforts we encourage will fail, and the cycle will continue.

In this part the options for prevention of malnutrition and its consequences will be considered. The importance of care in which all levels of society are engaged—from the affected child to public leadership—is stressed.

18

Problem of Changing Food Habits: How Food Habits Are Formed

Robert J. Karp, MD

The titles for this chapter and the next were chosen consciously as an homage to Margaret Mead, who wrote *The Problem of Changing Food Habits* for the War Department in 1943, and to Jean L. E. Ritchie who chose the title for a chapter in her now classic book, *Learning Better Nutrition* (1968). Many of the issues they presented are appropriate for today's poor in America. But there is a difference. The poor today are surrounded by the wealthy, and the world of wealth presented via the television and other mass media begs to be imitated. But Mead with prescience warned us to be wary of the consequence of having the poor imitate the rich. She wrote that while "an arbitrary balanced diet would be superior to the meals habitually eaten by the worst fed third of our population, there is a danger that the conventions of a balanced meal may be established at the higher income levels will sift down as 'style' to the lower income levels without the necessary knowledge to see that the meal is really balanced" (Mead, 1943).

Adjustments in diet that make sense and are sound at higher income levels are not so among the poor. The process for changing food habits was seen as different for the "worst fed third"—those we now call "the disadvantaged" (Wilson, 1988).

Early in the text (chapter 4), we described a food culture of chronic poverty that is as conservative as any indigenous food culture. Paul Rozin (1977) uses the term "neophobic" to describe the stabilizing and new food-rejecting qualities of a food culture. This chapter and the subsequent one provide information needed to undo the food culture of chronic poverty and replace it with one better adapted to poverty—a food culture that feeds children nutritious foods at a reasonable cost.

People are quite adept at putting together the oddest combinations to create a cuisine. The scientific tools of sociology and cultural anthropology as sciences are not adequate to describe totally how food habits actually change. Who could predict, as Rozin and Schiller note (1980), that Mexicans would combine chocolate and chilies to create a mole sauce unique to their culture? We can only describe what we see, as in the observations on a food culture of chronic poverty, and perhaps predict how changing phenomena in the society at large could affect food availability. We will only know how an individual responds to new choices when more stringent research methodology is developed.

Three concerns for this chapter are (a) children eat what they like (the influence of biology on food selection); (b) children like what they eat (the influence of learned preferences or culture); and (c) children eat what their families can afford to feed them (the influence of economics). Unanswered questions to be considered include the influence of micronutrient deficiencies—iron, calcium and zinc—on the mouthing behavior leading to lead poisoning and the effect of fetal alcohol exposure directly on taste and preference.

Sanjur (1982) said that food culture exerts a "locus of control" in food selection. Because none of the major influences can be isolated from one another, we will conclude the chapter with an approach to ethnicity that combines biology, culture, and economics. Four of the major ethnic groups in the United States will be described under the heading "Using Ethnicity to Break the Cycle of Poverty." This will be addressed by nutritionists who are active in the communities described.

CONSEQUENCE OF CULTURAL ISOLATION

In a story for children written more than 50 years ago, Andre, a French boy of the 17th century, is brought by his parents to a colony on Lake Champlain. Andre is befriended by a boy from the Ojibwa tribe of Native Americans. The life of the family is difficult. They clear the land, build cabins, and cut the wood needed to keep warm during the long New France winter. The families expect to live that first year on cooked game meat and cereal grains brought over on their ships. As winter passes, the colonists fall ill. They are tired and weak with aching muscles, bruised bodies, and bleeding gums. "We know about this," said Andre's new friend. He gives Andre tea made from the needles of the white pine tree to drink, and Andre is cured. The disease was scurvy; the cure was ascorbic acid (vitamin C) leached from the pine needles. The message of the curing tea is then passed to all the settlers, and they survive.

There is another story, one of nonadaptation and extinction. The Viking settlers in Greenland did not prepare fish in the same way as their Inuit (Eskimo) neighbors. By stewing whole cod fish and skimming the oil off of the top of the pot as a delicacy, the Inuit took in ample vitamin D to prevent rickets. By gutting the fish and discarding the innards—including the liver—the Europeans deprived themselves of a nutrient essential for their survival.

An important difference between the two stories is that the Vikings, unlike the French settlers, were socially isolated from Native American neighbors, who had several thousand years of experience in the far north. An epic legend of the Vikings from that time tells of the finding of an Inuit family stranded on an ice flow. As Rockwell Kent (1935) retells the story, the Vikings took the skrals (a pejorative term for the Inuit), cut off their arms, and fed them to the whales. It is no surprise that Greenland Inuit legend recalls the capture and killing of the last families of Vikings with pleasure rather than telling a story of shared traditions allowing for mutual survival.

These two stories encapsulate the dilemma of the disadvantaged poor. Survival of minorities depends on positive interaction with the dominant society, the judicious use of simple nutritious foods and condiments, and an ecology of food production and distribution that gets these foods to those who need them most. But, as Paul Rozin writes, "The major problem in world nutrition is to get people to eat foods that their culture rejects" (1975). This is the problem addressed in the present chapter.

CHILDREN EAT WHAT THEY LIKE: INFLUENCE OF TASTE IN CHANGING FOOD PREFERENCES

Children do eat what they like (Kare & Beauchamp, 1984, 1985). An understanding of how and why foods are liked or disliked is essential in planning a healthful diet that will be accepted by children. In a food culture influenced by poverty and *not* retaining elements of traditional ethnic cultures (see chapter 4), children are offered a limited selection of foods, and salt, sweet, and oil are the predominant tastes and flavors. This represents a "food culture of chronic poverty" that has characteristics analogous to those of more traditional cuisines (E. Rozin, 1983; P. Rozin & E. Rozin, 1977).

The perceptions of taste and flavor, have unique neural pathways and metabolic systems that are under the influence of neuroendocrine hormones. The reception, however, of a nerve impulse signaling a combination of tastes and flavors is not the same as the perception of taste or flavor (P. Rozin, 1990; Bartochuk, 1979). "Perception," writes P. Rozin, "is a behavioral term; it is not a mechanism but rather a description of behavior" (1990). It is certain that individuals experience taste and flavor of foods differently according to the social environment in which the food was first encountered and subsequent exposure. As Dr. Wachs notes (chapter 2), all environment is experienced differently based on biologic and sociocultural differences.

Biologic constraints to the effect of exposure will be addressed first. These include descriptions of (a) the intermediary steps between exposure and experience and (b) the influence of nutritional status and hunger on taste and flavor perception.

Exposure and Experience

The pathways between the tongue (first contact for taste) and the ethmoid plate (first contact for flavor and smell) and the receiving centers in the brain are quite complex. For taste, chemical substances eliciting primary sensations of sweet, salt, sour, bitter, and perhaps "hot" stimulate cells located on the tongue, for the most part, and on the palate, to a lesser extent (Kare & Beauchamp, 1984, 1985; Kare & Mattes, 1990). The cell impulses are transmitted to the brain stem for processing and then to cerebral centers. For flavor, receptors in the ethmoid plate sense the presence of volatile substance, much as in a gas chromatograph, again sending the stimuli to be received in the cerebral centers.

Genetic factors also influence taste perception. The difference between those who find saccharin to be an acceptable substitute for sugar and those who find saccharin to have an unacceptable aftertaste seems to be genetically determined (Bartochuk, 1979). Phenylthiocarbamide (PTC) is a substance thought to be bitter at low concentrations by some people, but is not recognized at all or only at high concentrations by others. PTC tasting is more common in populations exposed to bitter chemically analogous goiteragens (Bartochuk, 1979), suggesting the involvement of taste as protection in the evolutionary process (P. Rozin, 1975).

The four basic flavors are generally experienced as pleasurable by a child in the order sweet, salt, sour, and bitter (Kare & Beauchamp, 1984, 1985). The sensation of hotness is appreciated through pain receptors on the tongue and in the mouth, and is a learned taste preference for adults in some, but not all, cultures. Newborn infants like sweetened water; they smile and coo after a taste from a bottle. They are neutral to salt solution, but during the first year of life, their appreciation grows to a clear preference (Beauchamp, 1987). Infants grimace and turn away from sour and bitter. Mexican and Indian parents inevitably witness the pained response of an infant who accidentally tastes the families' favorite chilies and curries. Yet, after weaning and before adolescence, the favorite sour, bitter, and hot foods of a family also become the favorites of the children (P. Rozin, 1975).

The response to sweet is considered a protective mechanism for the infant so as to promote an appreciation of mildly sweet breast milk and, after weaning, calorie-containing foods. P. Rozin (1975, 1990) suggests that bitter foods are rejected because when our ancestors moved about the planet looking for new habitat, there was no easy way to distinguish between toxic and nontoxic bitter alkaloids. The biologic block slowed acceptance until humans could observe the response of animals to feeding and themselves to small tastes. Bitter foods are for the most part condiments rather than essential, though coffee and tea consumption suggest how important the contrast of bitter and sweet (plus some caffeine) is to food appreciation. Alternatively, as suggested by Beauchamp (personal communication, 1991) the ingestion of sweet should be considered a positive evolutionary imperative in that sweet foods contain energy, vitamins, and minerals (Logue, 1986).

The positive perception of sweet has been corrupted by the sweetening of potentially harmful products such as medicinals for children. Additionally, foods are sweetened to make them acceptable for commercial sale and use by children. Cereals and other traditional foods are sugared to make them more palatable. In some instances (e.g., the product Froot-Loops) so much sugar is added that the nutritional density (the ratio of nutrient value to caloric content) falls below levels acceptable to permit calling the product a food (Guthrie, 1978).

Public policy has had modest success in protecting families from these practices, but more effort is needed from the health care community. All families need to be educated to use safety precautions with medicines. Presweetening cereals provides far more sugar than sweetening at the time of use, and the purchase of these products should be strongly discouraged.

It is the responses to salt and sour that provide the greatest insight into the development of taste preferences. By 6 months of age, a child shows a positive appreciation of mildly salted water of a similar magnitude as the response to the mild sweet flavor (Beauchamp, 1987; Beauchamp et al., 1990). An early hypothesis was that the infant shows a learned response to early exposure by the parent to foods containing salt. Beauchamp examined the taste preferences of infants who were never exposed to salt and showed that this response is not learned (1987). Rather, the infant has a developmental appreciation of salt provided from the environment. The hypothesis is that the major evolutionary influence on taste preference is the long experience humans have had as essential vegetarians. In the purely vegetarian diet, consisting mostly of cereal grains, sodium balance is precarious. Humans are capable of conserving sodium with negligible intake. At very low levels of intake, however, the response to low levels of sodium concentration in or on food is heightened. A nonconsumer of salt will recognize and appreciate a low-sodium solution with gusto. Humans seem to have a "salt stat" in that a continued high consumption dulls the taste for low-level consumption and requires a higher level for the salt content to be appreciated.

Salting, and to a lesser extent souring (pickling), of food was an important discovery. It enabled the transport of food and the preservation of food for periods of scarcity such as between harvests or over the winter. Populations accustomed to high-salt foods continue that preference even when there is no biologic need. Salt-pork and salt-fish are staple foods for Americans from the south and Caribbean and Mediterranean peoples even when fresh, refrigerated, and frozen fresh foods are available. At the fast-food "burger/chicken" outlets in the African-American and Caribbean community near Kings County Hospital in Brooklyn, customers are asked, "Do you want extra salt?" on their already heavily salted purchases. As Ingelfinger notes (chapter 13) on preventing hypertension, this pattern of consumption has a significant negative effect on health.

But, as Beauchamp has shown (1987), all is not hopeless. A short period, 4 to 6 weeks perhaps, of sodium restriction allows a resetting of the "salt stat" so that lower concentrations of sodium would be experienced as saltier than the original baseline of acceptability (Beauchamp et al., 1990). Moreover, sodium ion on the surface of a food stimulates the taste receptor as well as much higher concentrations of sodium within the food. Thus fresh or frozen unsalted foods that are flavored at the time of consumption will have lower sodium content but equal or more salt-stimulating effect than canned or presalted foods. A similar "coating" phenomena probably accounts for the reduction in sugar or other sweetener used at the point of consumption. An essential need then is to encourage a substitute for the highly salted, non-nutritional, so-called junk foods consumed by many children and adults. This problem is not unique to the poor and disadvantaged.

A special vulnerability of poor children, with a heightened salt appetite or enhanced salt preference, is the possible consumption of lead-containing substances in the environment during the period of resetting the salt stat. As Beauchamp and Engelman (1990) note, depletion of minerals, in general, lead to an enhanced appetite for salt; "there are no specific tastes for other minerals and, in nature, salty tasting substances are almost always associated with other minerals."

Nutritional Status and Experience

It is important to ask if micronutrient levels influence taste and flavor perception. Kare and Beauchamp (1984, 1985) report the influence of vitamins A, B_6, B_{12}, nickel, copper, iron, and zinc deficiencies on perception of taste. Of these, iron and zinc require further comment in that disadvantaged children in the United States are affected by iron deficiency (chapter 9), and zinc depletion is associated with growth retardation (chapter 7). In infants, zinc deficiency is associated with fetal alcohol exposure (chapter 10). The contribution of sodium deficiency to taste perception has been noted earlier.

Zinc As it Affects Taste and Growth

Animal studies suggest that zinc deficiency is associated with "hypoguesia," a decreased taste perception. In elderly humans, zinc deficiency has been shown to impair the ability of dyorphin, an endogenous opiod, to promote feeding (Morley, 1988). This may reflect disturbance(s) anywhere in the pathways contributing to taste perception. However, in the absence of zinc deficiency, zinc replacement does not restore taste to the elderly.

In the study of growth and zinc in southern Ontario by Gibson et al. (1989), described in chapter 10 increased height velocity and caloric intake were found with zinc supplementation in those boys with reduced hair zinc levels. This one study suggests an impact on taste perception. The authors reported a higher pre-supplementation recognition threshold for salt in the reduced hair-zinc boys as compared to controls.

An additional variable is alcohol consumption and its effect on zinc metabolism, growth and possibly taste perception. As discussed in chapter 10, alcohol exposure in utero is associated with an embryopathy of FAS and with decreased body zinc, but the taste perception of FAS children has not been studied. A concern for subtle effects of FAS should be considered in subsequent studies of growth retarded children.

These studies, taken as a whole, suggest that we do not have all information we need to assess zinc nutriture. Perhaps "normal" measures of zinc in blood does not represent adequate zinc available at the intracellular level for metabolic functions essential for taste perception or, with respect to children, for growth (Solomons, 1988).

Iron, Calcium, Sodium, and Lead

It is imperative to repeat a comment from chapter 9 in a discussion of why children seeking divalent cations, might end up with lead poisoning. "Though lead should not be in the environment of any child, it is in the environment of many disadvantaged children." The first step in preventing lead poisoning is to end exposure of children to lead.

In 1959, Lanzkowsky suggested that deficiency in iron leads to a subconscious craving for divalent cations, which expresses itself in pica and, where lead is available in the environment, lead poisoning. In studies conducted among children with concomitant pica and iron deficiency, consumption of nonfoods ended with iron replenishment (Crosby, 1976; Lanskowsky, 1959). Studies attempting to link a heightened taste perception and preference for divalent cations, including both lead and iron, for children with iron deficiency have been inconclusive. Snowden (1977), in studies with rats, showed that the effect of calcium and zinc deficiency was stronger. He concludes that lead pica is a general response to mineral deficiencies—a position supported by Beauchamp and Engelman (1990).

Clinically significant lactose intolerance is an unlikely occurrence among young children—those under 18 months of age—in any racial or ethnic populations. By 5 years of age, however, 29% of black American children—with a lesser percentage for children of Western European ancestry—are lactose intolerant to the point of limiting their intake of dairy products (see Scrimshaw & Murray, 1988 for a comprehensive review of this topic). This decrease in calcium intake has, as a consequence, better absorption of lead (Mahaffey, 1981) and the potential consequence of heightened preference for substances containing lead.

CHILDREN LIKE WHAT THEY EAT: INFLUENCE OF CULTURE ON CHANGING FOOD PREFERENCES

We all begin life in utero, where nutrients are presented to us through an umbilical vein devoid of qualities that could be described as flavorable or preferred. After birth, the newborn has preferences, but they are only expressed in the circumstances of laboratory study. It is the nature of mammalian species (mama = breast) to feed infants their own milk. Although some differences do occur in the flavor of mother's milk, infants throughout the world from the time of antiquity have been fed a fairly uniform substance. Even at weaning, there is a similarity in the bland, high carbohydrate "beikost" (weanling foods) fed to small children. By age 8, however, adult food preferences seem well established. The child is fully acculturated (P. Rozin, 1990). He or she "likes what he eats" (Lewin, 1943).

We use powerful discriminatory abilities to distinguish perceived differences in food, to enjoy a new experience, and to reject the odd or unfamiliar. Food flavor, the aroma of a food, labels a food culture (E. Rozin, 1983). Taking a walk through any city, visiting delicatessens or markets, a person could know immediately where he was. An Italian or Greek "deli" would have the aroma of olives and various cheeses. A German or Hungarian deli would smell of sausages and the characteristic sweet spices of Central Europe such as paprika and dill. The reader who has experienced the pleasures of these foods is about to put down the book to look for at least one of the foods mentioned. But without experience, this is just a listing of unknown experiences, as foreign, uninteresting, or disgusting as the Eskimo custom of skimming and eating the cod's liver oil off a pot of boiling fish. Would any reader, other than a native of the far north, frequent a market where raw blubber and fermented, frozen meats were sold?

"Physical availability," wrote Lewin (1943), "is not the only factor which determines availability of food to the individual." "Cultural availability," meaning recognition that a product or substance is in the category of food, is of equal importance.

Rozin and Fallon suggest three broad categories of influences on a mother as she chooses food for her child (1981). She first asks, "Will my child like this food?" Here the academic distinction between the child liking what he or she eats, or eating what he or she likes is obscured by the mother's commonsense desire to give the child an acceptable food and having him or her like it. Although taste is stated as the cause for "liking," the sense of taste will be blended with the sense of flavor in the assessment of likability.

Second, a mother asks, "Will this food satisfy my child?" Foods that are filling and have no untoward affects, such as nausea or bloating, will be offered regularly. Awareness of intestinal upset is one of the major causes for food rejection (Rozin & Fallon, 1981). The milk rejection of many black families may reflect the consequence of lactose intolerance. Similarly, the consumption of beans and legumes may cause a gassiness. If there are common episodes of gastroenteritis, foods consumed just prior will be associated with the upset. At times enteritis is from bacterial growth with food spoilage where refrigeration or clean water is not available or not used.

Finally, a mother asks, "What do I know about this food?" Long-term health effects, social consciousness, and religious taboos also affect selection. Currently in the United States, we are discouraging the consumption of butter, lard, and other saturated fats and cholesterol for reasons that have little to do with gustatory satisfaction or the ability to make a pie crust—best made with lard. As discussed in chapter 14, excess restriction for the sake of preventing coronary heart disease can be harmful to the child. Finally, the information used may be incorrect as in the false belief that iron fortified formulas are associated with constipation.

Some beliefs must be respected absolutely. A committed vegetarian would respond to the offer of a meat meal with the same sense of disgust as most Americans have to the offer of fried slugs and worms. A sense of contamination makes these "meals" unacceptable. In this way, a substantial minority of Americans observe the biblical proscriptions against consumption of pork, shellfish, and the mixing of milk and meat. By contrast, some food associations are very powerful and positive, such as the foods consumed at a church picnic or Fourth of July barbecue, the turkey and stuffing at Thanksgiving, the ham at Christmas or special foods consumed by Moslems in the evenings during Ramadan, and by Jews at the Passover Seder and the subsequent week.

It seems clear that infants begin life with a minimal list of foods that they will not eat, but children develop into adults with the same fixed preferences as their parents. Thus, disadvantaged children are at risk for developing the food culture of chronic poverty when parents have this pattern of nonpreparation of foods to be consumed in social isolation. It is necessary to define the places at which intervention and prevention are possible.

Table 18.1 shows suggestions derived from Rozin and Fallon to affect food choices as would be applied to disadvantaged children (1981). A comprehensive set of suggestions, consistent with specific food cultures (ethnicities) of disadvantaged children are presented at the conclusion of this chapter.

TABLE 18.1 Suggestions to Affect Food Choices

Primary Influence	Course of Action
Will this food be liked?	Mask the flavor with preferred substances Since pizza (Italian food flavor) is the most universally accepted food in the United States, putting a mix of oregano, black pepper, garlic and tomato sauce on new foods will generally render them familiar.
	Encourage family eating and 'meals' and reinforce the importance of mother-child-family interactions around food
Are there consequences?	Teach food preparation skills and hygienic principles. Consider lactose or other intolerances.
What does the mother know?	Do not be fanatical about long term effects. Most importantly, it is essential to respect deeply held beliefs.

Do Children Have an Instinctive Ability to Select a Healthful Diet?

A much-quoted study by Davis (1928) suggested that over a period, when healthy toddlers are given free choice of foods they chose a nutritionally balanced, calorically adequate diet. Davis was well aware of the limitations of her work. Only three children were studied, and none of them had ever been exposed to the supersweetened foods now commonly available to children.

Recently, Birch et al. (1991) evaluated the intake of 15 children, 2 to 5 years of age, given free access to a varied supply of foods for 6 separate days. Twice as many calories as needed were made available to the children as a variety of nutritious foods. (Only one food item offered in a day was of low nutritional value.) There were wide variations in caloric intake through the day, but total daily caloric intake was fairly constant and not excessive. This suggested to Forbes (1991) that making foods freely available without compelling food consumption lessens the risk for obesity in young children.

All of the children in the Birch study were from homes where the parents were highly educated. Thus, these optimistic findings may not apply to the children from disadvantaged homes, where diets may contain almost 50% of calories from fat and sweetened snacks are commonly offered—the foods of chronic poverty. The warning from Mead (1943)—be wary of applying observations made of the well-off to the very poor—comes to mind.

CHILDREN EAT WHAT THEIR FAMILIES CAN AFFORD: INFLUENCE OF FOOD COSTS ON CHANGING PREFERENCES.

Children eat what their families can afford. As discussed in chapter 5, economic factors will predict in part the prevalence of undernutrition. Which form the malnourishment takes depends on the interaction of the food culture of the community and the economic system in determining the cost of food. Engels's phenomenon—as food costs rise, foods characteristic of higher earnings disappear from the table—governs, to a great extent, the nutritional quality of food choices (Karp et al., 1978; Karp & Greene, 1983). Poor families seek to provide the most energy at the least cost. When food selection narrows sufficiently, micronutrients disappear from the diet and malnutrition ensues.

Figure 18.1 shows a mathematical model of the Engels's phenomenon. A family of five (two adults and three children) has an expected caloric intake of 10,000 calories per day. The U.S. Department of Agriculture Low Cost Food Plan (LCFP) costs $12 ($0.12/100 calories) and is one third of daily income ($36 for this family) at the poverty level—point A.

An increase in income of $3 a day would result in almost $1 going for food. The nutritional value of the food obtained at $0.13/100 calories will be somewhat better—as much as can be expected on an income of $39 a day for a family of five—point B.

Supplemental food plans work in two ways (Karp, 1985). Consider the worth of $5 of food supplementation. First, the foods provided are of a high nutritional value. Second, the family is relieved of the responsibility of purchasing a substantial part of their daily caloric need. If the family of five receives WIC for an infant, school feeding programs for two older children, and food stamps for the entire family, the aggregate provision is of 4,000 calories. This leaves 6,000 calories to be purchased for the same $12 a day and foods costing $0.20/100 calories such as fresh fruits, vegetables, and lean meat can be purchased. This increases the nutrient value of the remaining part of the daily diet and equalizes intake to that of middle income families—point C.

In theory, with bare-subsistence income, nearly 100% of free income will be spent on food. At the other extreme, with unlimited income, the caloric limit for intake is reached, and food consumption, in and of itself separate from entertainment, is a rather low percentage of income. For middle- and upper-class Americans with disposable incomes of greater than $15,000 per year, food expenditure runs below 15% of income. At the poverty level, however, a minimal expenditure for food,

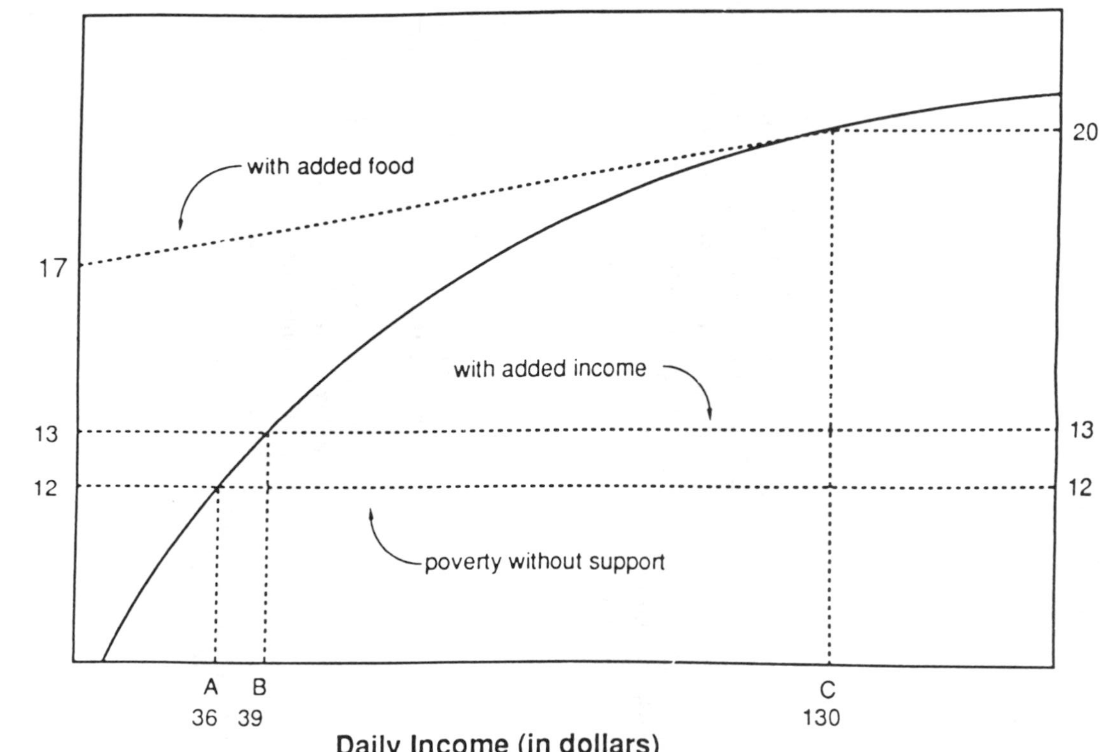

FIGURE 18.1 Engels's law with and without supplementation for a family of five consuming 10,000 calories a day.

Adapted from Immink (1982); Karp et al. (1978); Karp and Greene (1982).

as set by the government, is 33% of income. In fact, the very poor will spend substantially more than one third of their income on food. One estimate of poor people's income, given the list of other essentials, suggests that there is not disposable income to be used for nonessential items when income is below 300% of the poverty level (Who Can Afford Health Care?, 1989). Yet, in some states, our nation's single most effective program, the Supplemental Feeding Program for WIC spends all of its allotted funds with only 50% of eligible families (185% of poverty level income) served (Stockman, 1987).

One prejudice against the poor is that the savings from food go for drugs, alcohol and tobacco. Careful evaluation shows that, on the contrary, there is a full supplemental (saved income goes for food) effect for WIC and 50% of savings from food stamps are used for supplementary food purchases (Price, West, Shier, & Price, 1978). The school feeding programs, for unknown reasons, result in higher than supplementary expenses by the family (Mauer, 1984) as well as an increase in overall improvement in nutrient intake (Hanes, Vermeersch, & Gale, 1984). Long (1991) has found ". . . . that somewhat less than one-half of each additional dollar of NSLP benefits is used by households for supplemental food expenditures, while all of each additional SBP benefits is allocated to such expenditures."

Early versions of prudent diets (see chapter 14) stressed the consumption of rice and beans with smaller quantities of animal products than usually found in commonly consumed high-fat diets. The newest version of these diets, with five to nine portions of *fresh* fruits and vegetables per day, are inconceivable for poor families without such commitments. (See Figure 18.2.)

Simply stated, without supplementation, poor families are highly vulnerable to malnutrition however well they harbor their resources. With adequate income support and supplementation, however, the overwhelming majority of poor families will compensate for poverty and provide their children with nutritious food. As Berg (1982) writes, "The extra amount spent on food will result in an improvement in the quality of the diet for the family. With a better diet in the family as a whole, individuals within the family, including the children will have better nutritional status."

SUMMARY

Economic improvement enables the better nutrition required for disadvantaged children to break out of the cycle of poverty. Recommendations cannot be made, however, without considering the indigenous

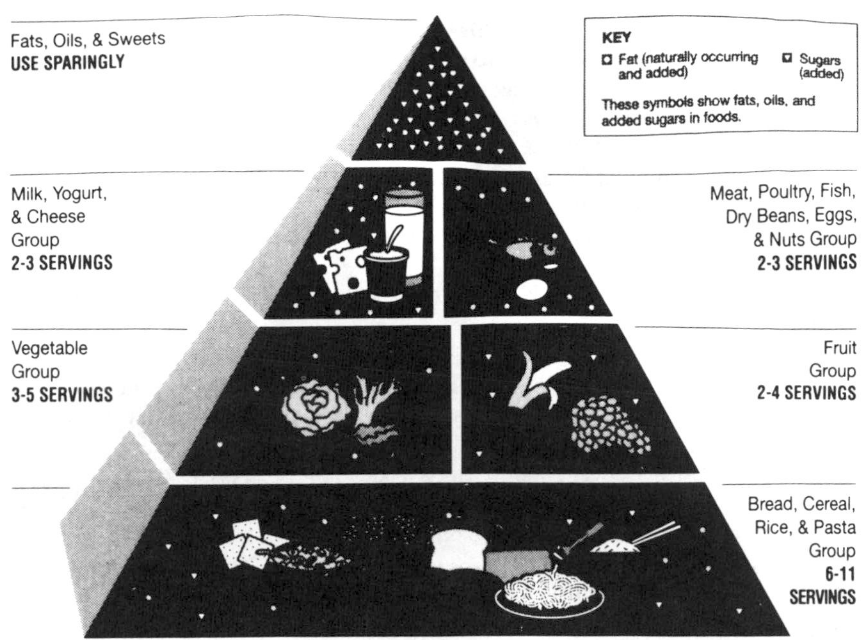

FIGURE 18.2 Food guide pyramid: A guide to daily food choices.

food culture(s) of families affected by poverty. The next chapter provides comments of five dietitians actively working in communities where people from the major ethnic groupings in the United States live.

ACKNOWLEDGMENT

The help of Tracy Burgess, MD, in preparation of this chapter is greatly appreciated.

REFERENCES

Bartochuk, L. M. (1979). Bitter taste of saccharin related to the genetic ability to taste the bitter substance 6n-propylthiouracil. *Science, 205*, 934–935.

Beauchamp, G. (1987). The human preference for excess salt. *American Scientist, 75*, 27–33.

Beauchamp, G. K., Bertino, M., Burke, D., & Engelman, K. (1990). Experimental sodium depletion and salt taste in normal human volunteers. *Am J Clin Nutrition, 51*, 881–890.

Beauchamp, G., & Engelman, K. (1991). High salt intake: Sensory and behavioral factors. *Hypertension, 17*, 176–181.

Berg, A. (1982). Food preference as a determinant of food behavior. In D. Sanjur (Ed.), *Social and cultural perspectives in nutrition* (pp. 123–146). Englewood Cliffs, NJ: Prentice-Hall.

Birch, L. L., Johnson, S. J., Andressen, G., et al. (1991). The variability of young children's energy intake. *NEJM, 324*, 232–235.

Crosby, W. H. (1976). Pica: A compulsion caused by iron deficiency. *Brit J Hematology., 34*, 341–342.

Davis, C. (1928). Self selection of diet by newly weaned infants. *Am J Dis Child., 36*, 651–679.

Forbes, G. B. (1991). Children and food—order amid chaos. *NEJM, 324*, 262–263.

Gibson, R. S., Vanderkooy, P. D. S., MacDonald, A. C., et al. (1989). A growth-limiting, mild zinc deficiency in some southern Ontario boys with low height percentiles. *Am J Clin Nutrition, 49*, 1266–1273.

Guthrie, H. A. (1978). Concept of nutritious food. *J Am Diet Assoc, 71*, 14.

Hanes, S., Vermeersch, J., & Gale, S. (1984). The national evaluation of school feeding programs: Program impact on dietary intake. *Am J Clin Nutrition, 40*(Suppl.), 390.

Immink, M. D. C. (1982). Purchasing power and food consumption behavior: how poverty level is defined. In D. Sanjur (Ed.), *Social and cultural perspectives in nutrition* (pp. 91–122). Englewood Cliffs, NJ: Prentice-Hall.

Johnson, S. C., Burt, J. A., & Morgan, K. J. (1981). The Food Stamp Program: Participation, food costs, and diet quality for low income households. *Food Tech, 35*, 58.

Kare, M. R, & Beauchamp, G. K. (1985). The role of taste in the infant diet. *Am J Clin Nutrition, 41*(Suppl.), 418–422.

Kare, M. R., & Beauchamp, G. K. (1984). Taste, smell and hearing. In M. J. Swenson (Ed.), *Duke's physiology of domestic animals* (pp. 742–760). Ithaca: Cornell University Press.

Kare, M. R., & Mattes, R. D. (1990). A selective overview of chemical sense. *Nutrition Rev, 48*, 39–48.

Karp, R. J. (1985). Increasing the intake of nutrients while reversing the Engels phenomenon [letter]. *JAMA, 254*, 3178.

Karp, R. J., & Greene, G. W. (1983). The effect of rising food costs on the occurrence of malnutrition in the United States: The Engels phenomenon in 1983. *Bull NY Acad of Med, 59*, 721.

Karp, R. J., Fairorth, J., Kanofsky, P., et al. (1978). The effect of rising food costs on hemoglobin concentrations of early school age children. *Public Health Reports, 93*, 456.

Kent, R. (1935). *Salamina*. New York: Harcourt, Brace.

Lanzkowsky, P. (1959). Investigation into the aetiology and treatment of pica. *Arch Dis Childhood, 34*, 140.

Lewin, K. (1943). Forces behind food habits and methods of change. In *The problem of changing food habits* (Bulletin of the National Academy of Science, No. 108). Washington, DC.

Logue, A. W. (1986). *The psychology of eating and drinking.* New York: Freeman.

Mahaffey, K. (1981). Nutritional factors in lead poisoning. *Nut Rev, 39*, 353–362.

Mauer, K. M. (1984). National evaluation of school nutrition programs: Program impact on family food expenditures. *Am J Clin nutrition, 40*, 448–453.

Mead, M. (1943). *The problem of changing food habits.* (Bulletin of the National Research Council, No. 108). Washington, DC: Food and Nutrition Board, National Academy of Science.

Morley, J. E. (1988). Trace elements. In J. E. Morley (Moderator), Nutrition in the elderly. *Ann Intern Med, 109*, 890–904.

Nutrition Review. (1986). Zinc and fetal alcohol syndrome: Another dimension. *Nutrition Reviews, 44*, 359–360.

Price, D. W., West, D. A., Shier, G. E., & Price, D. Z. (1978). Food delivery programs and other factors affecting nutrient intake of children. *Am J Ag Econ, 60*, 619.

Ritchie, J. A. S. *Learning better nutrition.* (1968). Rome: Food and Agriculture Organization.

Rozin, E. (1983). *Ethnic cuisine: The flavor principle cook book.* Brattleboro, VT: Stephen Greene.

Rozin, P. (1990). Acquisition of stable food preferences. *Nutrition Rev., 48*, 106–113.

Rozin, P. (1977). The use of characteristic flavorings in human culinary practice. In C. M. Apt (Ed.), *Flavor: Its chemical, behavioral and commercial aspects* (pp. 101–127). Boulder, CO: Westview Press.

Rozin, P., & Fallon, A. E. (1981). The acquisition of likes and dislikes. In J. Solms & R. L. Hall (Eds.), *Criteria of food acceptance: How man chooses what he eats* (LWT-Editionen: Reviews in Food Science and Technology, No. 6, pp. 35–48). Zurich: Foster Verlag.

Rozin, P., & Rozin, E. (1976). The selection of foods by rats, humans and other animals. In J. S. Rosenblatt, R. A. Hinde, E. Shaw, & C. Beer (Eds.), *Advances in the study of human behavior* (Vol. 6). New York: Academic Press.

Rozin, P., & Schiller, D. (1980). The nature and acquisition of a preference for chili pepper by humans. *Motivation and Emotion, 4*, 77–101.

Sanjur, D. (1982). Social and cultural perspectives in nutrition. Englewood Cliffs, NJ: Prentice Hall.

Scrimshaw, N. S., & Murray, E. B. (1988). The acceptability of milk and milk products in populations with a high prevalence of lactose intolerance. *Am J Clin Nutrition, 48*, 1988–1159.

Sebrell, W. H. (1955). Biographical essay: Joseph Goldberger. *Journal of Nutrition, 55*, 3–12.

Snowdon, C. T. (1977). A nutritional basis for lead pica. *Physiology and Behavior, 18*, 885–893.

Solomons, N. (1989). Zinc and copper. In M. E. Shils & V. Young (Eds.), *Modern nutrition in health and disease* (6th ed., pp. 238–262). Philaelphia: Lea & Febiger.

Stockman, J. A. (1987). Iron deficiency anemia: Have we come far enough? *JAMA, 258*, 1645–1647.

(1989, summer). Who can afford health care? *Health Advocate, 161*, 3.

19

Problem of Changing Food Habits: Reaching Disadvantaged Families Through Their Own Food Cultures

Maudene Nelson, MS, RD,
Rosalind Bowser, RD,
M. Yvonne Jackson, RD, PhD,
Borinquen Lugton, RD,
Rene Murray-Bachmann, RD, and
Patricia Giblin Wolman, EdD, RD,
with summary by Robert J. Karp, MD

Culture and ethnicity influence rather than control the behavior of individuals, with the exception of food selection. Here, as Sanjur correctly points out, culture asserts a locus of control that cannot be ignored if there is to be a healthful adaptation of diet by the disadvantaged of any ethnicity (1982). This chapter describes the effect of chronic poverty on the food culture and thus the nutritional well-being of poor families in the United States.

The food cultures of five groups—Native Americans, African-Americans, Hispanics, and Caribbean peoples, and rural poor whites—are described, but the examples drawn from their experiences could be applied to anyone. While paying respect to the generations of wisdom that gave rise to a food culture, this chapter examines the behavioral, social, and environmental factors that alter and, at times, erode the survival effects of food culture. We consider the pronounced effects of chronic poverty on food culture and the subsequent nutritional well-being of children. The concluding summary is a set of principles applicable to all disadvantaged families, regardless of race or ethnicity, in our society.

HOW FOOD CULTURES DEVELOP

Every time we eat, we exhibit behavior that identifies our food culture. The choice to eat fish as opposed to pork, rice as opposed to potatoes is made with implicit rules. A food culture is that set of behaviors relating to food that are characteristic of a particular social culture. Food culture is taught by formal and informal means. The household member in charge of procuring the family's food—usually a woman, who is herself in a culturally defined position—sets before the family explicit lessons on what constitutes a culturally appropriate meal and how it must be served. The relative quantities of various foodstuffs, the degree of piquant, texture, and mixtures are explicit. As described by Barker (1982), exceptions to the rule that the process of food selection precedes cultural imprinting is very rare in traditional settings.

Although there is a finite number of foods available to humans (using categorical distinctions such as legumes, milk products, grains, etc.), the variety of food cultures is impressive. As noted in chapter 4 the four characteristics that distinguish a food culture are (a) the basic substances of the diet, (b) the flavors used to give character, (c) the methods of preparation, and (d) the social setting for eating. Of these, flavoring most distinguishes the cuisine of one culture from another (E. Rozin, 1983; P. Rozin & E. Rozin, 1976).

The role of the food culture is to ensure the survival of its members. It must meet psychological and social needs as well as provide sufficient nutrients. The ability of people to make appropriate changes in their food culture in the face of social, economic, physiological, or geographical changes is a true test of survival. To use a construct drawn from the work of Maslow (1954), food is needed initially for survival.

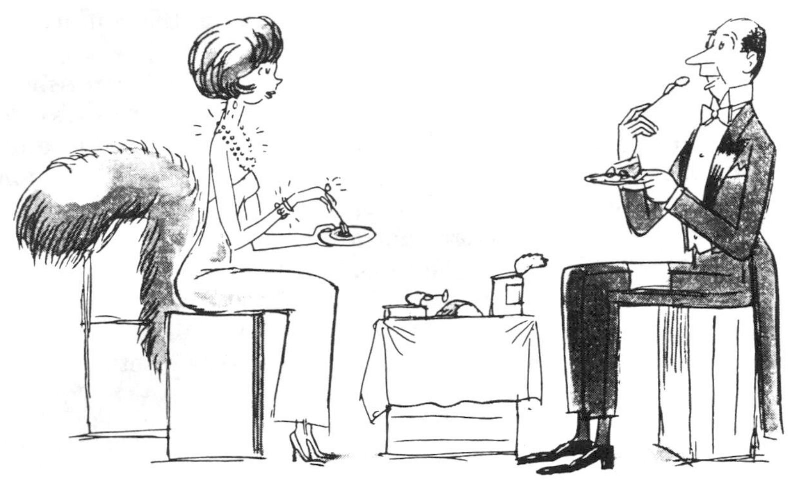

Attempts to rise in the social scale may have an unfortunate effect on nutrition because there is not enough money for both socially desirable items and good food.

FIGURE 19.1

From Ritchie (1968). Reprinted with permission.

Once a subsistence level is reached and food can be stored for the future, there is security. At that time, a unique food culture is created allowing members of a group to develop a sense of belonging or group identification that is symbolized by their food choices. Within the group, however, stratifications occur that allow food choices to be used to achieve status. What one eats and with whom states one's real or desired status in his or her own culture as shown in Figure 19.1. In a mature food culture, the individual, secure about the availability of food and satisfied with his or her position in the society, achieves what Maslow calls self-realization. The individual is now free to explore the food of other food cultures.

Poverty and Loss of Cultural Pride

One has to question why the richest agricultural country in the world fails to feed its own people adequately. In 1967, the Citizens Board of Inquiry into Hunger and Malnutrition in the United States found hunger in Appalachia, on Indian reservations, in urban ghettos, and in backwoods areas of the South. Previously, the United States government had surveyed hunger in 32 foreign countries but not at home (Cross, 1987). As will be shown by Nestle (chapter 24), we know what to do, but we will not do it wholeheartedly. The Food Stamp Program, the Special Supplemental Feeding Program for WIC, the various programs under the Child Nutrition Act (e.g., school lunch, school breakfast, summer feeding program) have had beneficial effects on the nutritional status of children. But the persistence of the effects of hunger and malnutrition among people in chronic poverty raises a question that other pernicious factors influence access to food. Part of the answer to the question "Why does persistent malnutrition exist?" may be the ability of a particular food culture to adapt and continue to nourish its people.

As documented by Karp in chapters 4 and 18, limitations on buying power affects people's ability to procure an optimal, not to mention adequate, diet. But this explanation may be too simplistic. A persistently low economic status affects the survival aspects of a food culture (i.e., basic substances of the diet, the methods of preparation, and the social setting in which food is eaten), because it compromises the emotional fabric of the members of the culture. As Rosen notes in chapter 25, mainstream society in the United States devalues the culture of poor ethnic minorities through social isolation and the use of stereotypic negative images. Social behavior, including food behavior, is affected. Traditional ways of eating, which are generally nutritious, are demeaned and often abandoned or altered in ways that diminish nutitional value.

As long as the basic substances of a food culture are there, the methods of preparation, food flavors, and social setting can be modified, and the people will survive. But when faced with the need to change, basic foods are the least likely to be replaced. Any food culture whose basic foods cannot be obtained will be devastated. The potato famine in Ireland in the 1800s is a case of a people at a near-subsistence level of existence severely hurt by the loss of basic foods from their diet.

DISTINGUISHING THE FOOD CULTURE

In the sections of this chapter, we consider how the food cultures of poorer groups put them at special nutritional risk in a dominant society that does not necessarily provide for the needs of those who are different. We list the four characteristics of food culture from Rozin and Rozin, and follow with a discussion of the pressures of chronic poverty on these groups who are most at risk for malnutrition.

Basic Substances

As with all food cultures, the foodstuffs that are readily available in the environment will be the staples. The "three sisters"—corn, beans, and squash—are grown together and prevail as a self-sustaining nutritional/agricultural system used by Native Americans throughout the Americas. The high nitrogen needs of corn are helped by the nitrogen-fixing bacteria of the beans. The bean vines, in turn, use the corn for support. The squash (or any plant from the pumpkin family) wanders about, its broad leaves shading the ground, protecting its "sisters" by slowing the evaporation of moisture from the soil. Nutritionally, the complemented proteins of the grain and legume, the complex carbohydrates available in the three vegetables, the vitamin C, beta-carotene, and trace minerals provide a nutrient-dense system. Most Hispanic food cultures contain some version of the "three sisters."

But not all basic substances from which meals are provided are considered equally. The genesis of the phrases "high on the hog" and "whole hog," reflect the prevalence of pork in the diet in the southern United States. As noted earlier, the better off one became, the fewer knuckles and feet were eaten and having a "whole hog" was the mark of a wealthy household. These concepts are not unique to the culture of African Americans; in fact, what is referred to as "soul food" is characteristic of rural poor Southern people, both black and white.

The rural poor eat less dark green vegetables, less deep yellow vegetables, less citrus fruits and juices, but more potatoes, than their urban counterparts. People living in urban areas spend 24% more of their food budget on fruits and vegetables than those living in rural environments (and more of their food money on food away from home) than those living in rural areas (*Family Economics Review*, 1987). This difference is most probably due to the lack of transportation and cold storage outside of cities. Rural poor families, who do not own cars, can travel to a grocery store at best once or twice a month. They are more likely to subsist on foods that can be stored in minimal space such as canned foods, rice, peanut butter, dried peas and beans, Kool-Aid, iced tea, and other nonperishable items (J. Shotland, et al., 1987).

Home-grown food has been, in the past, an important source of food for rural populations, but those who live in cities tend to romanticize rural life and underestimate the resources needed to grow foods to be used as staples (rather than supplements) to the diet (see Figure 19.2).

The contemporary Native American diet is a combination of indigenous and traditional foods plus commercially available fresh and processed foods. Wild game and fish, where available, provide important sources of food. Wild fruits, berries, roots, and greens are highly valued foods, but scarce in many areas. The symbolism of food often determines food acceptance. Among the Navajo, for example, meat and blue cornmeal are considered "strong" foods, while milk is a "weak" food. The Seminole Indians of Florida consider meat a food that gives one

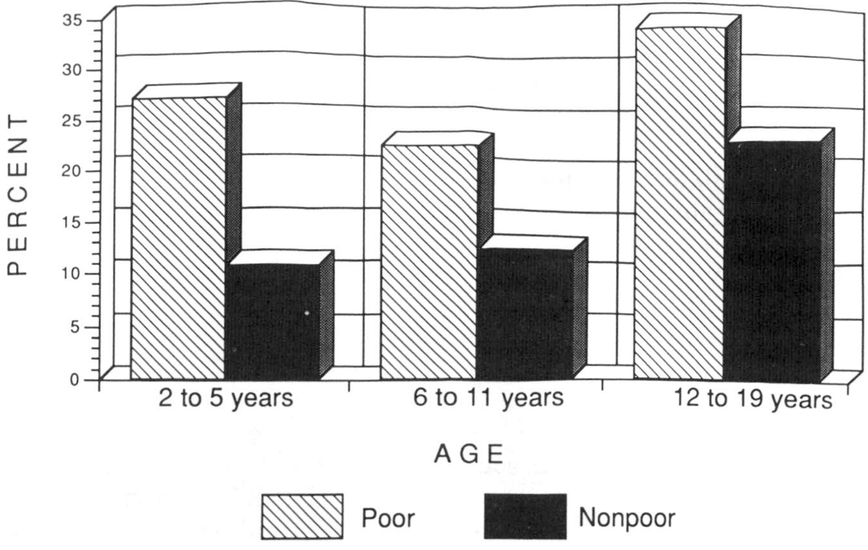

FIGURE 19.2 Percentage with less-than-weekly intake fruit and vegetables rich in vitamin C.

strength, while vegetables are not highly regarded, and patients are often confused when counseled to substitute vegetables for calorie-dense foods. "Significantly," writes Joos (1980), "there is no Indian [Seminole] word for 'vegetables,' and in translation, the Indian word for vegetable is synonymous with 'weeds.'" Thus the health professional counseling the consumption of vegetables may be recommending an inedible substance.

Methods of Preparation

Traditional families living in rural areas have prepared food from home-grown supplies. This included home canning of fruits and vegetables and home curing of pork. A cast iron skillet, roasting pan, rice pot, and a large pot for boiling were standard kitchen apparatus. The main method of preparation was frying of steaks, chops, fish, and eggs. The fat of choice for both frying and baking was lard, though eventually, hydrogenated vegetable shortenings came into use. Leafy and ocher green vegetables and tubers were boiled—always with pork flavoring. Fruits and yams were often eaten stewed or candied. Hence, a significant amount of sugar (white and brown) and salt were commonly used. All of these traditions have been brought to the city and form the basis of the African-American diet.

In traditional Caribbean and Latin American homes, foods are cooked largely on top of the stove (i.e., boiling, simmering, stewing, and frying). White rice is usually cooked in boiling salted water with fat (lard or oil) for flavoring. In Puerto Rico, the rice at the bottom of the pot generally browns and becomes crisp. This "pagao" is very popular. A mainstay of the diet is the hearty soup (sancocho) that efficiently and nutritiously simmers noodles, vegetables, and meats, and other ingredients as needed or available to feed a large family. This is referred to as "pot" cooking in the African-American community.

Food Flavors

Black Americans and rural southern whites have traditionally used sweeteners liberally. Jellies and jams were popular. Yams were usually candied, and many high sugar desserts and soft drinks are appreciated.

Food flavors are still dominated by salt and salted pork products—even as the flavoring agents have more than doubled in price and are of little or no nutritional value. Engels's phenomenon, "as food costs rise, food selections narrow to those providing the most energy at lowest cost," is illustrated by rural southern families, which, when times are good, can consume all cuts of the pig—both high and low on the hog.

When these families move to the urban north and have to support themselves on low-wage employment, the cuts of meat, if put together, would not add up to a whole hog. Instead of getting the rich hocks, loin, and shoulder of the pig, excessive fatty cuts, such as jowls and knuckles are eaten. The lean parts are replaced by the fat, salt, and flavor of the pig. As a result, young black children in the United States have higher intakes of total fat and cholesterol than white children during their early years of life (Nicklas et al., 1987).

Among the Caribbean peoples, a characteristic flavoring is "sofrito," a minced blend of garlic, green bell pepper, onion, coriander leaves, and small round sweet peppers (ajiles dulces) sauteed in pork fat or cooking ham. Another is a commercial preparation called "adobo," a powdered spice blend consisting of salt, garlic, oregano, and black pepper. A low-salt adobo can be made by changing the proportions of the ingredients. A yellow coloring is imparted to foods by adding a small flower bud, annatto (achiote), to hot lard or oil during the cooking.

In general, Hispanics are fond of sweet flavors. The abundance of sugar cane makes it comparable with fruits as a snack food to the detriment of dental health.

Latin American foods are characteristically spicy and salted heavily. Salsa, a tomato, hot pepper and onion relish, and chili sauces (made with a variety of yellow, green, and red chili peppers) dominate the food flavors of Latin America. The frequent use of cocoa is seen in Mexico as mole sauce, a mixture of cocoa and hot peppers. Cocoa is also widely used to flavor milk and is more prevalent in this diet than the diets of other ethnic groups. Guacamole, a sauce based on avocado, onion, and chilies, is particularly popular in Mexico.

As noted in chapter 18, the process of change to a healthful diet must be in the context of foods with familiar flavors. These traditional flavors, plus that of Italian-American, the most popular American cuisine (tomato sauce, garlic, oregano, and black pepper) can be used to modify less-than-nutritious diets in families.

Social Setting for Eating

There is a vision that many of us carry along in life. Meals, we remember, were served family style, and the head of the household sat at the head of the table. Adults, particularly when company was present, had first access to the food. At times, in poorer families, this resulted in children having a limited variety and quantity of foods. Children would eat after or apart from adults if the social setting deemed their presence secondary. In most cases, however, bounty as well as scarcity would be fairly distributed. And the family was together.

This contrasts dramatically with the food culture in chronic poverty. A family is often a young mother, her small or school-age child or children, and a relatively young and inexperienced grandmother, who may also have borne her children quite young. Their meal preparation may be the work of the grandmother, though the mother is responsible for feeding her small child. Familiar staple foods may be prepared in the home at least once a day, but the family-style dinner table may not exist. When an experienced adult is not available to prepare traditional staples, many convenience foods are used in their place. Boxed macaroni and cheese, carry-out Chinese food, fried chicken or pizza, fast-food combinations, packaged cookies, and ready-to-eat cereals are a few examples. Commercial inducements, such as advertising on television, diminish the importance of home-prepared foods.

Instead of a family breakfast and evening meal, foods are brought in and warmed or not available at all throughout the day. Obesity results when some members of the household take every opportunity to eat what's around; "meals" turn into continuous eating. The signals and lessons on satiety and overall balance of food stuffs are missing from the dining experience. The rituals of blessing the food and adjusting intake to the entire meal's offering (i.e., leaving appetite for dessert or remembering that having a heavy lunch means that dinner will be light) are observed with less frequency.

These changes are not unique to the poor. They are part of a national trend, but, as with everything else that affects the poor, the harmful results are exaggerated, and the gain is minimal. The skill and wisdom of preparing and serving a meal is losing ground among all Americans including the poor. The diminished quality of the diet of the disrupted food culture of those children living in chronic poverty reflects an inability to maintain good nutrition in the face of a changing national food culture based on convenience. Successive generations of the poor have lost the pleasure of food in the family home to the detriment of the nutrition and nurturing of children.

SOME SPECIAL CONCERNS

The nutritional problems of disadvantaged children are too great to be addressed through the application of a general formulation, however well constructed that may be. There are other issues to be considered, some of which are noted subsequently.

Consequence of Poverty in the Caribbean

Special concern must be raised for the poverty and endemic undernutrition that exists in parts of the Caribbean, especially Haiti. The Haitians have witnessed, and perhaps experienced, conditions that are close to famine. This is true, to a lesser extent, of people emigrating from other parts of the Caribbean.

A typical child's diet in Haiti would be

Breakfast: A slice of bread and coffee with milk
Lunch: Fried chicken or beef with rice, beans, bread, coffee, and milk
Dinner: the same as breakfast

If the family's financial status is extremely depressed, the evening meal will be omitted. Although the Haitians continue to be poor after emigrating to the United States, the Haitian immigrant finds it easier to earn money and purchase food of various kinds. The family will have access to an abundant supply of their native food in local markets as well as the opportunity to purchase some of the high-fat and high-carbohydrate foods consumed by people of all ethnic backgrounds in the United States (e.g., fast-food chicken and burgers).

Thus, it is not uncommon for these children, in the United States, to have a weight for age and a weight for length or height above the 95th percentile with the parents thinking that this is "just right." After having been so nutritionally deprived in their own land, the Haitian mother has a tendency to overcompensate for the previous lack.

Nutritionists will find great resistance to attempts at weight control. Mothers often say, "She cries all the time that she is hungry, so I just give her what she wants." Grandmothers at home are particularly resistant to diet recommendations made to the mother in the clinic. As discussed in chapter 12, it is essential to examine family dynamics. As Bradley will show in chapter 20, the most important person in the family (the "pivotal person") must consider the changes valid before they are accepted.

White and Poor

In 1987, according to the U.S. Bureau of the Census, 10.5% of whites and 33.1% of blacks were living in poverty with the greater proportion of the black poor living in cities (*Family Economics Review*, 1989). Whites make up 75.1% of the nonmetropolitan poor population, but only 52.3% of the urban poor are white. The rural poor are less educated and are more likely to live in two-parent households than are their urban counterparts. The number of white, rural poor has grown during the 1980s because of the loss of family farms and of jobs affiliated with the oil and automobile industries (Shotland et al., 1987). The "new poor" are individuals who worked all of their lives, often accumulating substantial assets, but who now must accept positions at minimum wage. Although these are families in which both parents work, they are often forced to sell off their assets and eventually ask for assistance from food banks to feed their children. The new poor are unlikely to ask for assistance from federal programs even though they are eligible under the law. For example, in Kansas, only 5% to 15% of the eligible poor receive food stamps (Shotland et al., 1987).

In examining the diets of rural, white poor families, it is assumed that (a) poverty leads to undernutrition, (b) food choices will be influenced by the culture of the family, and (c) it is possible to get an adequate diet on a poverty income if one possesses essential coping skills. Each of these assumptions contain a part of the truth; no one of them describes the whole.

The food culture found in many rural white communities in the United

States separates foods that are healthful or "good for you" from those that are enjoyable. Children are trained to eat foods that are nutritious only to get the reward food. "You can't have dessert unless you eat your vegetables" is a common admonishment of parents. Unfortunately, when children learn to divide food into "good foods" that are eaten for health and "bad foods" that are eaten for pleasure, they begin to view nutritious foods as undesirable and eat them only under duress (Mead, 1943).

Poverty is also a great influence on the diet as discussed earlier in this chapter. Therefore, the rural poor must be vigilant about their food purchases, and home gardening should be encouraged as an excellent source of vegetables that can be eaten fresh and canned, or frozen for use all winter. But gardening requires one or more strong adults with the time and energy left after a day at work to put into physical labor. Gardening is also risky, entailing the investment of precious food dollars in seeds, equipment, and fertilizer for food that can be eaten only a few months or, should bad weather, pests, or other losses intervene, never. Canning and freezing require investment in jars or containers, and assume the availability of a range and freezer.

Concerns for Native American Children

In many Native American cultures, food has great religious and social value. Food is an integral part of numerous celebrations, and is a main attraction at feast day celebrations, powwows, and religious ceremonies. Hospitality, which includes serving food, is a serious obligation. It is socially and culturally unacceptable for a guest to refuse food offered at these occasions. Likewise, it is unacceptable not to serve food to any visitors. Some families will exhaust their scarce food supplies to meet these social obligations. The family will then go without food until resources become available for obtaining food.

As noted in chapter 10, there is a continued concern for the use of alcohol among many, but not all, Native American groups. The prevalence of FAS on different reservations in the Southwest varied between 1 in 97 to 1 in 749 in the early 1980s (May, 1986). It has been estimated that 1 in 20 Sioux Indian women living on the reservations in South Dakota has the potential for giving birth to an infant with FAS (Peterson et al., 1984). As discussed in Chapter 10, children with FAS do not grow well. They experience feeding problems, and adjustment to solid foods is often difficult. The nutritionist must play an active part in the community to prevent FAS.

Dental caries are also an important problem among Native American children associated with soft-drink consumption baby-bottle tooth decay (BBTD). In a recent study, 72% of a Navajo Indian sample in

Arizona and New Mexico and 55% of a Cherokee Indian sample in Oklahoma exhibited some level of BBTD (Broderick et al., 1989).

It is always hazardous to make generalizations about Native Americans because there are numerous differences both among tribes and within a tribe. There are, however, certain common considerations that should be applied in the nutritional counseling of Native Americans whether they live in urban or rural areas, or on reservations, whether they have acculturated to the dominate society or not.

Family. An understanding of family structures is exceedingly important when planning and conducting prevention and intervention strategies. Most Native Americans place very high value on the family—to be poor in the Indian world is to be without family. Native Americans do not distinguish between close and distant relatives. A relative is a relative. Native American infants and young children frequently have multiple caretakers within the extended family. Compliance with health regimes is increased if the extended family members are involved in developing and implementing the care plan.

Native American children are raised in a permissive atmosphere and are allowed to make independent decisions at an early age. A child is free to decide when to eat, the kinds and amounts of food to eat, what to wear, when it is time for bed, and so on. This can result in irregular eating and sleeping times.

Because children make independent decisions, it is vital that they are included in planning prevention and intervention programs. An adult caretaker normally will not tell a child what to eat or not eat. Even a child 4 or 5 years of age should be dealt with directly with an adult assisting the child in carrying out the agreed-on strategy. For example, in evaluating the diet of a 6-year-old obese boy, you learn that he eats a large quantity of cookies each day. The two of you agree he will eat three cookies only after he has walked to and from his grandmother's house—a total of three miles. The role of the adult caretaker is to remind the boy of his agreement.

Individual. Traditional cultural values place great importance on respect and considerations for others. Discussing another person, even giving information about a family member for a medical history, may be considered interference or meddling.

Many Native Americans consider their inner thoughts and personal lives to be private and will avoid answering questions about what they consider personal matters. In the counseling situation this may appear as though the patient is uncooperative or indifferent.

Traditional Medicine. For years Native Americans have relied on traditional medicine healing to respond to the issues surrounding

TABLE 19.1 Navajo Translation of Nutrition Terminology

English	Navajo	English Translation
Nutrients	Iineiidziil	life/energy, power, strength food
Calories	Ch iyaandziil yolta	energy, power, strength/count of the body
Protein	Ats iistah bee no nise	in parts/by means of/it grows
Fat (food)	Bil ch iyaan ai inigii	grease that is made with foods
Fat (body)	Hak ah	body fat
Iron	Dil bii aziil	blood/within/that is particle
Calcium	Ats in bii aziil	bone/within/that is particle

Source: Navajo Tribal Food and Nutrition Services, 1987.

illness. In some Indian Health Service hospitals, medicine men are included in the health care delivery system. Diet is an integral part of traditional medicine. Herbalists prescribe special diets that eliminate certain foods for curing purposes. Ingestion of herbal medicines or foods with spiritual properties are used in many traditional healing ceremonies. Some foods, particularly fruits and vegetables, are forbidden while using some traditional medicine. Where corn is considered sacred, cornmeal is sprinkled on the floor around the bed of a hospitalized patient in a variety of curative ceremonies. Items believed to possess special healing powers, like juniper berries, may be placed on a patient's bedstand or hung on the bed.

Communication. Differences in language impede communication, as does lack of understanding of medical and nutritional terminology. Interpreters should be used to facilitate communications whenever necessary. However, misunderstanding can occur even with an interpreter. Some English words and concepts do no exist in Indian languages or are not easily translatable. The reverse is also true of some Indian words and concepts.

Nutrition terms are among the words that can be translated in a variety of different ways. Some tribes, like the Navajo, are developing new native words that describe nutrition terms rather than relying on the introduction of English words that would have to be learned by many people (Yazzi et al., 1987). Some of the nutrition terms developed by the Navajo Tribal Food and Nutrition Services (1987) are illustrated in Table 19.1.

In the absence of a systematically developed standardized interpretation of nutrition terms, the selection of an interpreter is vital. This suggestion is appropriate for families from any community, including those where English is the native language, because the meaning of a word or phrase to the speaker may have little relation to the meaning perceived by the listener.

RECOMMENDATIONS FOR ALL

As early as 1943, Margaret Mead warned that food habits should be changed without sermons, preaching or attaching moral values to specific foods. She said that children can learn to eat and enjoy nutritious foods simply by watching their parents eat and enjoy nutritious foods. But how do we teach parents to be good role models, if they did not learn it from *their* parents? Ethnic minorities—immigrants who arrive under conditions of poverty as well as groups of native poor people—face an even greater struggle to achieve an optimal diet. At times language difficulties or differences, even as minor as an accent, and the need to become acclimated present significant obstacles to obtaining necessary resources. Even in the best of circumstances it is difficult for people to reestablish or maintain cultural practices, including food culture, immediately after relocating.

Facing Difficult Truths

The stress on the food culture of relocating is not unique to immigrants. Poor people in the United States are more likely to move around than nonpoor, and poor blacks move 3 times more often than poor whites. All of the factors discussed in this section—poverty, lack of education, cultural isolation, and insecurity—as well as the additional obstacles of not having familiar foods readily available, impaired ability of families to prepare food in the traditional manner, having the social setting radically interrupted, in effect, sets the stage for nutritional compromise of the family. And children are the most vulnerable members of the family.

Change must be based on established eating patterns rather than trying to make drastic changes. Point out the beneficial components of the diet eaten by many poor families (e.g, dried peas and beans, grits, rice, greens, and potatoes). Health workers often assume that everyone should eat a "typical American diet" and make suggestions to "Eat more fish, chicken and fresh vegetables." Although a diet consisting of only rice, beans, and grits would indeed be unhealthy, lack of variety is the problem, not the foods themselves. Poor families could continue to use familiar, inexpensive foods as the mainstay of healthful eating patterns with encouragement and direction for adding variety to their diets. Common sources of nutritious foods of reasonable cost (within

TABLE 19.2 Sources of Nutrients: Foods Costing at or below $0.12/100 Calories

VITAMIN A—greens: beet, collard, dandelion, mustard, etc., kale and spinach, carrots, sweet potatoes, winter squash, pumpkin, rutabagas, livers (high in cholesterol), eggs, prunes and watermelon.

VITAMIN C—white and sweet potatoes, cabbage, turnips, rutabagas, okra, lima beans, green peas, and greens: beet, turnip, collard, dandelion, mustard, kale and all fresh fruits.

PROTEIN—eggs, dried peas and beans, peanut butter, dry skim milk, wild game, fish, including tuna and sardines, red meat and livers (high in cholesterol), cornbread, crackers and pasta.

IRON—All of the protein list plus greens (when consumed with meat and vitamin C-containing foods)

CALCIUM—All dairy products plus bony fish (sardines) and greens

the $0.12/100 calories recommendation for the Low Cost Food Plan) are listed in Table 19.2.

Respecting Cultural Diversity

Understanding and respecting cultural diversity is a major challenge to health care practitioners. Health workers should work with each disadvantaged family individually because all poor people (urban and rural, white, black, Hispanic, Caribbean, Native American or the numerous ethnic groups not described individually) are not alike, though they may have characteristics in common. We must be aware of our own health beliefs, attitudes, and values to bridge successfully cross-cultural gaps between the provider and the family. Listed subsequently are techniques and approaches that address some of the challenges posed in providing meaningful, relevant health prevention and intervention for all ethnic and cultural groups.

1. Recognize and respect each patient's health care beliefs. Determine the client's perceptions of health, illness, and disease. Ask about health customs and practices; listen, and correct for your cultural biases. For all persons with strongly held beliefs, the best approach is to integrate traditional and scientific medical practices.
2. Learn about the community's cultural food behaviors. Ask patients about traditional foods, food preparation methods, and meal patterns. Learn what is available in the food markets, from food assistance programs, and what foods are grown locally, harvested, or hunted. Find

out what are the unique food and preparation methods used by the community. Encourage traditional food ways by helping patients integrate these foods into their diets, especially for ceremonies and celebrations. As much as possible, serve traditional foods in hospitals; include their use in food demonstrations. Become aware of the traditional medicine diet prescriptions and food taboos to minimize conflicts with biomedical diet prescriptions.

3. Develop culturally relevant nutrition programs to teach self-help skills. Food as a therapeutic intervention is an integral part of traditional beliefs in all cultures, although it is most prominently related to medicine in Native American and Caribbean cultures. Build on diet therapy's high status in traditional medicine, and incorporate it into biomedical nutrition counseling.
4. Develop family support. Learn about the family support systems. Involve family members whenever possible.
5. Adjust all patient-encounter situations to the pace and literacy level of the patient. Do not hurry, and take time to ensure patient understanding.

Helping Families to Develop Coping Skills

To make the most elementary changes in nutritional practices, most poor householders need basic coping skills including (a) abstract thinking ability (understanding that sound nutritional practices today will have an impact on health tomorrow); (b) mathematical skills (required for comparative shopping); (c) food preparation skills (buying the least expensive foods requires being able to prepare and cook them properly); (d) food storage skills (purchasing fresh requires an understanding of how foods spoil); (e) literacy (lengthy forms must be completed for eligibility for supplemental food programs); (f) transportation (shopping and federal or private food program offices are often distant from home); and (g) strong moral fiber (an ability to maintain human dignity in a system that denigrates individuals and assumes fraud on the part of the recipient).

But above all else, health workers need to get involved in improving legislative and regulatory policies for food and nutrition programs on the federal, state, and local levels so that nutritious, culturally acceptable foods are available to all groups and families.

SUMMARY

Well established food cultures of poorer communities in the United States have faced relatively abrupt changes. The children of these cultures are most often the first to exhibit symptoms of malnutrition. Throughout this text, various authors have cautioned against too great an emphasis on culture as a control of, rather than a response to, environment and experience. Labeling of behavior, as defined by culture or race/ethnicity, is a highly prejudicial act. Assumptions made because of physical appearance, mode of dress, speech patterns, or mannerisms prejudge a person based on common assumptions about a group—most of which are false. As with socioeconomic status, the dimensions of ethnic groups are too broad to make assumptions about any single member.

While paying respect to the generations of wisdom that gave rise to a food culture, we have examined the behavioral, social and environmental factors that alter and, at times, erode the survival effects of food culture. From the analysis contained in these two chapters (18 and 19), however, we have constructed the means by which both tradition and good nutrition can be maintained.

REFERENCES

Barker, L. M. (Ed.). (1982). *The psychobiology of human food selection.* Westport, CT: AVI.

Broderick, E., Mabry, J., Robertson, J., et al. (1989). Baby bottle tooth decay in Native American children in Head Start centers. *Pub Health Rep, 104,* 50–54.

Cross, A. T. (1987, August). Politics, poverty and nutrition. *Journal of the American Dietetic Association, 87,* 1007–1010.

Family Economics Review. (1989). Money, income and poverty status of families. *Family Economics Review, 2,* 20–21.

Joos, S. K. (1980). Diet, obesity, and diabetes melittus among the Florida Seminole Indians. *Florida Science, 43,* 148–150.

Maslow, A. H. (1954). *Motivation and personality.* New York: Harper & Row.

May, P. A. (1986). Alcohol and drug misuse prevention program for American Indians: Needs and opportunities. *J Stud Alcohol, 47,* 137–195.

Mead, M. (1943). Dietary patterns and food habits. *J Am Diet Assoc, 19,* 1–5.

Navajo Tribal Food and Nutrition Services. (1987). Translation of nutrition terminology.

Nicklas, T. A., Frank, G. C., Webbe, L. S., et al. (1987). Racial contrasts in hemoglobin levels and dietary patterns related to hematopoiesis in children: The Bogalusa Heart Study. *Am. J. Public Health, 77,* 1320–1323.

Peterson, L. P., Leonardson, G., Wingart, R. I., et al. (1984). Pregancy complications in Sioux Indians. *Obstet Gynecol, 64,* 519–523.

Ritchie, J. A. S. (1968). *Learning better nutrition.* Rome: Food and Agriculture Organization of the United Nations.

Rozin, E. (1983). *Ethnic cuisine: The flavor principle cook book.* Brattleboro VT: Stephen Greene.

Rozin, P., & Rozin, E. (1976). The selection of foods by rats, humans and other animals. In J. S. Rosenblatt, R. A. Hinde, E. Shaw, & C. Beer (Eds.), *Advances in the study of human behavior* (Vol. 6). New York: Academic Press.

Sanjur, D. (1982). *Social and cultural perspectives in nutrition.* Englewood Cliffs, NJ: Prentice-Hall.

Shotland, J., Kelly, P. B., Loonin, D. & Haas, E. (1987). Profiles of rural poverty: Facing barriers to the food stamp program. Washington, DC: Public Voice for Food and Health Policy.

Shotland, J., & Loonin, D. (1988). Patterns of risk: The nutritional status of the rural poor. Washington, DC: Public Voice for Food and Health Policy.

Yazzi, T., Hudson, W., Pelican, S., et al. (1987, July). Toward the divulgement of culture and language: Nutrition education messages for Navajo audience. Presented at the annual meeting of the Society for Nutrition Education, Denver, CO.

20

Nurturance and Nutrition

Joanne Bradley, PhD, EdD

There is no doubt that poverty is the "economic precursor" of malnutrition in children. Although poverty provides the material conditions for malnutrition, cultural and social factors interact with economics to affect the nutritional status of children raised in material disadvantage. That is, not all poor children are undernourished,. We are led, therefore, to ask, why do some poor children grow up well nourished, whereas other poor children do not?

It is necessary to consider the importance of maternal nurturance for childhood nutrition and explored what is known about nurturance as it affects nutrition. In trying to understand the complex nexus of social and emotional factors involved in shaping the mother–child relationship, we will look at those social factors that put mothers at risk for psychological depression, and we will explore the consequences of that depression for the health and welfare of their children.

NURTURANCE

Infants are born helpless and remain dependent on their parents for a long time. This dependence is purposeful, for the human infant requires a long period of nurturance to ensure that it thrives. Infants are dependent not only for food and physical care, but for *affectionate* care and attention (Klaus & Kennell, 1976). Nurturing behaviors include fondling, gazing, massaging, kissing, and making soothing sounds. Through these nurturing behaviors and nutritional satisfaction, the infant is reassured.

Nurturing is the process of guiding the child toward self-actualization and is an ongoing process. Throughout the child's lifetime, the strength and character of the nurturing process will influence the quality of all the child's bonds to other individuals including their own children.

Some women are simply overwhelmed by the burdens of poverty, the responsibilities of paid and unpaid work, and, quite often, the additional burdens of sexual and racial discrimination (Sidel, 1986). In response many suffer from moderate to severe psychological depression. That depression manifests itself in feelings of helplessness and hopelessness that often emotionally paralyzes a woman and interferes with her ability to care for herself or for her children.

NUTRITION

It is likely that the mother–child relationship is a central explanatory variable in the development of malnutrition among poor children. In their study of 9,000 disadvantaged urban children in Baltimore, Hepner and Maiden (1971) found a significant number of children (though not all) with growth failure, deviant laboratory values, and borderline or deficient cognitive and behavioral development. They found a significant correlation between the emotional-cognitive relationship between mother and child on the one hand, and the nutritional status of the child on the other. They concluded that the mother–child relationship was a "controlling factor" in preschool child nutrition, whereas "adequate 'mothering' is protective to the child under the combined stresses of rapid growth and low-quality nutrient intake, and (2) . . . inadequate 'mothering' precipitates malnutrition in the rapidly growing child even with more adequate, and more balanced nutrient intake."

There is a common, correct belief that abused children are likely to have parents who were abused when they were children. The statement in reverse, however, is *in*correct. Not all adults who were abused as children will continue the abuse in the next generation. Neither biology nor experience are destiny. The reason for that is explained by Freiberg, Adelson, & Shapiro (1987): "There are many parents who have themselves lived a tormented childhood who do not inflict pain on their children. These are parents who say explicitly, or in effect, 'I remember what it was like. . . . I would never let my children go through what I went through.' "

This research, among others (Cravioto & DeLicardie, 1972; Karp et al., 1984; Pollitt, 1975) presents convincing evidence of the importance of parental behavior to the nutritional well-being of infants and children, particularly among families whose poverty puts them at a material risk. But, having said this, we are immediately lead to ask why mothers of poorly nourished children are not responding to the physical and psychological needs of their children.

This question reframes our conceptual formulation from one in which the child's nutrition is the dependent variable and the mother's behavior the explanatory or independent variable to a formulation in which the mother–child interaction is seen as a consequence or outcome of some broader sociological process. A more adequate formulation must include a variety of factors that lead to the psychological depression in some poor women that in turn impairs their ability to nurture their children. Poverty and the responsibility for young children are among the most salient risk factors for depression among women. Thus the cycle of poverty turns on material conditions that place poor children at risk for malnutrition and their mothers at risk for psychological depression, also.

STRESS, DEPRESSION, AND THE INABILITY TO NURTURE

"Much of the stress in life," writes Belle (1982), "comes not from the necessity of adjusting to sporadic change [as is measured in life events checklists], but from steady, unchanging (or slowly changing) oppressive conditions which must be endured daily" (Dohrenwend et al., 1980). As shown by Belle, the most stressful area in poor women's lives is money, followed by parenting, living conditions, and intimate relationships. Significantly, those women who experienced more stressful and less supportive environments also experienced more symptoms of psychological depression. Yet stressed mothers expressed a great deal of care and concern for their children. Many recognized the problems they were having giving their children the care they needed within the trying conditions of their lives. Thus, interventions that address only the mother–child relationship without providing broad support for *all* aspects of mothers' lives will not be as successful in improving the well being of low income mothers or their children.

NURTURING THE NURTURERS

Intervention and prevention efforts can be seen as providing nurturance to those women whose responsibility it is to raise children within social and economic situations of deprivation so that they in turn can effectively nurture their children. It is clear that it is beyond the ability of many women to cope with the burdens they face, and intervention efforts must address these very real needs if they are to be successful. Education efforts (including the teaching of specific parental skills, information on nutrition, food preparation, etc.) must be culturally relevant and accessible.

"PIVOTAL PERSON"

Children are at risk of being poor, regardless of race, when raised in female-headed households. However, if they are black, they are at even greater risk of being poor (*Five Million Children*, 1990). It seems appropriate, then, to look at this population and suggest why some of these poor black children grow up well nourished and nurtured, and others do not.

The family as defined in the United States is understood as being a father and mother, and dependent children (nuclear family). The nuclear family is also considered primarily for child bearing and rearing, as defined by European standards. Black families reflect to a great degree the influence of their West Africa culture versus the more Western approach to child bearing and rearing. Standards and values in the family are handed down by what the black community calls "pivotal persons." These people operate as stable filters between the larger society and the individual. Although a pivotal person may be anyone in the child's immediate environment (aunt, uncle, minister, older sister, teacher, grandparent), he or she takes on the responsibility of educating the family and the children. The pivotal person is responsible for the socialization process within the black family, which includes teaching manners, morals, skills, and values. He or she provides an intergenerational continuity for black families (Bradley, 1989).

The identity and role of the pivotal person is implicitly understood among family members and quite often within the immediate community. Age, sex, or status of the family member does not necessarily play a role in the inheritance of this honor, but rather the ability to translate beliefs.

Poor families that include a stable pivotal person are more likely to have well-nourished and well-nurtured children (Karp et al., 1984). Understanding the role of the pivotal person can assist the health professional in several ways. Health care professionals working with poor families will find they can relate better to their patients if the pivotal person is somehow involved in decision making, for they make great allies for change. For the health care provider understanding the culture, values, and manners of their clients, as well as the role of the pivotal person, improves their chances of being successful in the health care treatment they recommend to their clients.

SUMMARY

Psychological and support services are needed to help poor mothers develop the cognitive and emotional resources to care for themselves and their children. These services should be given by providers familiar with the culture and, when possible, should include the pivotal person. However, therapy for low-income mothers must address the environmental stressors, mostly related to poverty, which contribute to women's psychological reactions.

REFERENCES

Belle, D. (1982). *Lives in stress: Women and depression.* Beverly Hills, CA: Sage.

Cravioto, J, & DeLicardie, G. (1972). Environmental characteristics of severe clinical malnutrition and language development in survivors from kwashiorkor and marasmus. In *Nutrition: The nervous system and behavior* (PAHO Scientific Publication No. 251). Washington DC: Pan American Health Organization.

Dohrenwend, B., Dohrenwend, B. S., Gould, M. S., et al. (1980). *Mental illness in the United States: Epidemiological estimates.* New York: Praeger.

(1990). *Five million children: A statistical profile of our poorest young children.* New York: National Center for the Study of Children in Poverty, School of Public Health, Columbia University.

Freiberg, S., Adelson, E., & Shapiro, V. (1987). Ghosts in the nursery: A psychoanalyic approach to the problem of impaired infant–mother relationships. In S. Freiberg, *Selected writings* (pp. 100–136). Columbus, OH: Ohio State University Press.

Hepner, R., & Maiden, N. C. (1971). Growth rate, nutrient intake and "mothering" as determinants of malnutrition in disadvantaged children. *Nutrition Reviews, 29,* 219–223.

Karp, R., Snider, E., Fairorth, J., et al. (1984). Parental behavior and the availability of foods among undernourished inner-city children. *Journal of Family Practice, 18,* 731–735.

Klaus, M. H., & Kennell, J. H. (1976). *Maternal-infant bonding.* St. Louis: Mosby.

Pollitt, E. (1975). Failure to thrive: Socioeconomic, dietary intake and mother-child interaction data. *Fed Proc, 34,* 1593.

Sidel, R. (1986). *Women and children last: The plight of poor women in affluent America.* New York: Viking Penguin.

21

Role of Schools and School Nurse

Jeanette Fairorth, EdD, RN, and Robert J. Karp, MD

The public school, an institution for all children, holds an inherent positive purpose and is mandated for use. Free public education is a relatively new phenomenon in the United States and in the world at large (Katz, 1976). Today, laws that require children to enter school by age 7 years and stay in school to age 16 years are uniform throughout the United States. The school stands between the family and the health profession, and may provide our best opportunity to reach disadvantaged children in their communities. The school nurse can be the crucial link.

Schools have a special place in the life of a disadvantaged child. People we know who have risen from abject poverty and torn families report consistently that it was in school where they found a supportive environment and a person who recognized their intelligence, diligence, creativity, and other worthwhile characteristics.

In this chapter, we consider the role of the school nurse in the identification and treatment of malnourished children, both educational and therapeutic, related to nutrition. Most important, we consider the contribution that school feeding programs have made to the well-being of disadvantaged children.

ROLE OF SCHOOL NURSE IN IDENTIFICATION OF MALNOURISHED CHILDREN

An important role for the school nurse has been to monitor the growth of children. The school nurse can use this information to identify children who are at risk for malnutrition. The school health service then serves as a means of entry into the disadvantaged family for the identification and treatment of malnourished children (Adobonojo, 1973; Karp et al., 1976).

Home Study

In communities that are economically disadvantaged, somatic growth at levels below the norm may be associated with poverty, malnutrition, and deprivation. As noted by Wachs, (chapter 2), it is the home situation, the microenvironment of the child, which has the greatest influence on the development of the child. The problem is: How does one obtain entry into the home?

In a health and nutrition project conducted in a North Philadelphia school, a medical evaluation of inner-city children provided us with the opportunity to investigate the growth of preschool siblings of those school children found to be minimally retarded in somatic growth (Karp et al., 1976). Each of the schools had a nurse responsible for health screening, providing general advice to children and teachers, communicating with local physicians, and record keeping. The Follow-Through program had a physician (R. K.) and a Public Health nurse (J. F.) who were available to support the school nurses.

The homes of all children in the at-risk group were visited by a home health aide who was active in the school program. All preschool children were brought into the school for evaluation, which included health history, examination, and measurements of height, weight, and hemoglobin level. In this study, we found that 14 (10%) of the 143 originally evaluated children were found to be at risk for malnutrition. Only 52 (28%) of the school children were identified as "well nourished"—having all measurements above the minimal acceptable levels defined for the study. Seventy-seven (62%) of the children originally tested had one or two of these measurements of somatic growth below the minimally accepted levels.

The "B" family was found to have no food available for consumption. There were two younger siblings in this family with measurements suggesting protein-energy malnutrition and iron deficiency. A significant association was found between being at risk for malnutrition and delay of entry into elementary school. Each of these findings suggests a role for the nurse in the identification of children with malnutrition and seeking help for malnourished children.

Assessment of Children in School: Case Study

Freddie P. was an 82-month-old boy with growth measurements at the 10th percentile for age and sex. He was doing poorly in the second grade, and he was placed in a combined kindergarten/first grade. Because he was close to 7 years old, he did not appear to be smaller than his classmates. At the time of the group assessment, Freddie was pointed out to medical students as an example of a kindergarten child with "appropriate growth." With adjustment of height and weight for age and sex, it was shown that he was substantially undernourished. Moreover, the height age, as shown in Figure 21.1 was closer to achievement levels than was chronological age.

With respect to the "P" family, our home investigation found an overwhelmed single mother who lived in an apartment with no furniture. A dietary history found Mrs. P. unable to prepare food. The only solids given to Freddie were cold cereal with milk. Mrs. P. was a kind, gentle, and concerned parent, but she had to be taught to make sandwiches with meat and peanut butter. With subsequent measurements, Freddie showed catch-up growth.

The "B" family identified in the formal study had more serious problems. This family had withdrawn from society, and the children were neglected. Help (intervention for neglect) for that family was sought from the Children's Protective Service Division of the Department of Public Welfare of the City of Philadelphia. For the other families in the study, and for the family of Freddie P., nutritional information and medical treatment were provided. These families were assisted in making application for supplemental food programs. Teachers were informed of their nutritional problems, and extra school lunches were provided.

LIAISON WITH THE COMMUNITY

The British have had a tradition of a home health visitor, which long predates their National Health Service. The home visitor is usually a registered nurse with training in public health. She arrives at the home of each newly born child in her district without regard to the income, education, or social status of the family. This removes the potential of social stigma from having a visitor. Her role in the health care team is to give comfort to the new mother and, at times, act as a liaison (for the health service) for families with special needs. This service

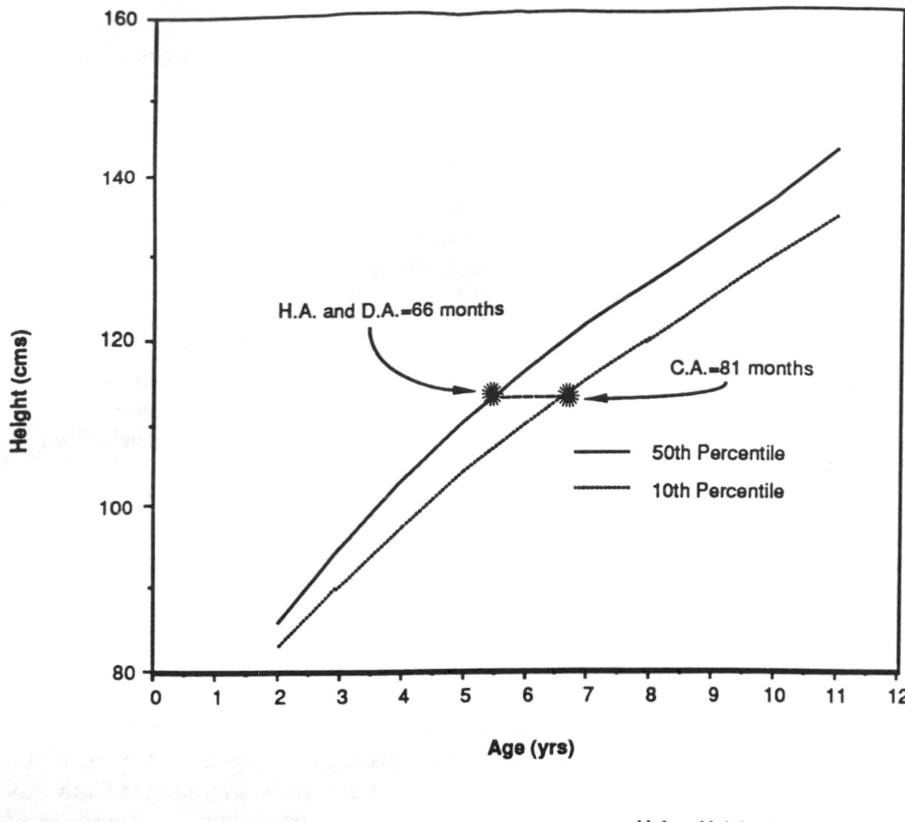

FIGURE 21.1 Note that height and developmental age are at about the same level and substantially lower than chronological age. Children with growth retardation appear to be well nourished when their growth failure and learning failure combine to place them in the school grade of younger children (see chapter 3).

is still in place in Great Britain and is used throughout the world. Henry Kempe (1973), a pediatrician actively involved in the prevention of child abuse, strongly recommended home health visits to at-risk children as an essential component of prevention.

Our own health visitor, Ophelia Mitchell, was a middle-aged woman whose grandson was a school student. Her effectiveness as a home visitor is exemplified in a study of families of iron-deficient children (Karp et al., 1974) where she gained the confidence of 67 of the 69 families to obtain entry into the home, complete the survey, and provide nutrition advice and iron therapy. Although administrative and political problems may seem overwhelming in school systems, we believe that an effective school-based health team requires a home visitor or community worker (Olds & Kitzman, 1990).

SCHOOL-BASED NUTRITION EDUCATION

School health programs have long been a part of public health programs in the United States. For nearly a century, school health programs have played a significant role in the control of communicable diseases by means of health inspections, immunization campaigns, and related activities (Pigg, 1989). Numerous evaluation studies of school-based nutrition education programs have demonstrated that when the education programs are implemented in classrooms, they produce positive measurable effects on children's and adolescent's knowledge of nutrition (Kalina et al., 1989). The effects on attitudes and behaviors are less consistent across the studies but are clearly evident.

Currently there is a movement under way to "bridge the gap between community and school health" (Green, 1988). This movement calls for the involvement of primary care health professionals in school health and nutrition programs. *School Health: A Guide for Health Professionals* (American Academy of Pediatrics, 1987) is a useful reference for health care providers interested in becoming involved in school health. Nader (1988) cautions that it is wise for health care providers, who become involved in school health, to distinguish between their roles as caregiver for a given child and as health consultant to a school.

Nader's approach, adapted to nutrition-related problems, suggests that a health professional (a) hold an in-service workshop (on obesity, perhaps) for school personnel, (b) advise the school board on the need for school breakfast, (c) assist the curriculum director with specific nutrition content, and (d) publicize and support school nutrition efforts with patients and parents. These are very different roles from that of the school physician or nurse providing health care directly to children.

Health care providers, who wish to work in school nutrition education, should be aware that several different groups are already involved in this endeavor. These include local Dairy Council units, Nutrition Education and Training Program coordinators, and cooperative extension agents, to name a few.

SCHOOL FEEDING PROGRAMS

The School Feeding Programs were established in the post–World War II years for two reasons: (a) to support farm income by providing a consistent market for American agriculture and dairy products, and (b) "to safeguard the health and well-being of the nation's children by providing them with nutritious food (Radzikowski & Gale, 1984).

Effect of School Breakfast

The unfortunate reality in the life of children from the poorest and most disadvantaged homes is to come to school hungry—without breakfast, and this may affect school performance (Pollit et al., 1978; Read, 1973). Because hunger is not a form of malnutrition, measures of nutritional status may be normal. A well-nourished child will have sufficient glycogen stores to maintain blood glucose levels for an overnight fast. During periods of fasting, there is a switch in metabolism to ketones produced in the liver, but this switch is not activated quickly. Thus, without early-morning glucose provision, the brain may not function effectively.

In a study in Jamaica, Simeon and Grantham-McGregor (1989) showed the synergism between missing breakfast and prior malnutrition on skills in language fluency, performing arithmetic tasks, and maintaining short- and long-term memory. Figure 19.2 shows an association between problems likely to lead to learning failure and breakfast deprivation in children with prior malnutrition. "The control group was not adversely affected in any of the cognitive tests when breakfast was omitted. . . . In contrast, the previously malnourished and the stunted groups were adversely affected in fluency (a measure of generation of ideas and motivation) and coding (visual short-term memory). Relative to the control children they were also adversely affected in arithmetic" (Simeon & Grantham-McGregor, 1989).

The well-nourished children seemed less affected. The study is unique in that it delineates a group of children who had a history of malnutrition. The authors suggest that the nutritional deprivation had affected the state of central nervous system arousal required for the children to achieve in learning situations.

"Clearly," they write, "the association is complex and performance depends not only on the state of arousal but also on the type and difficulty of the task and the nature of the subjects. It is possible that malnourished children have levels of arousal different from those of con-

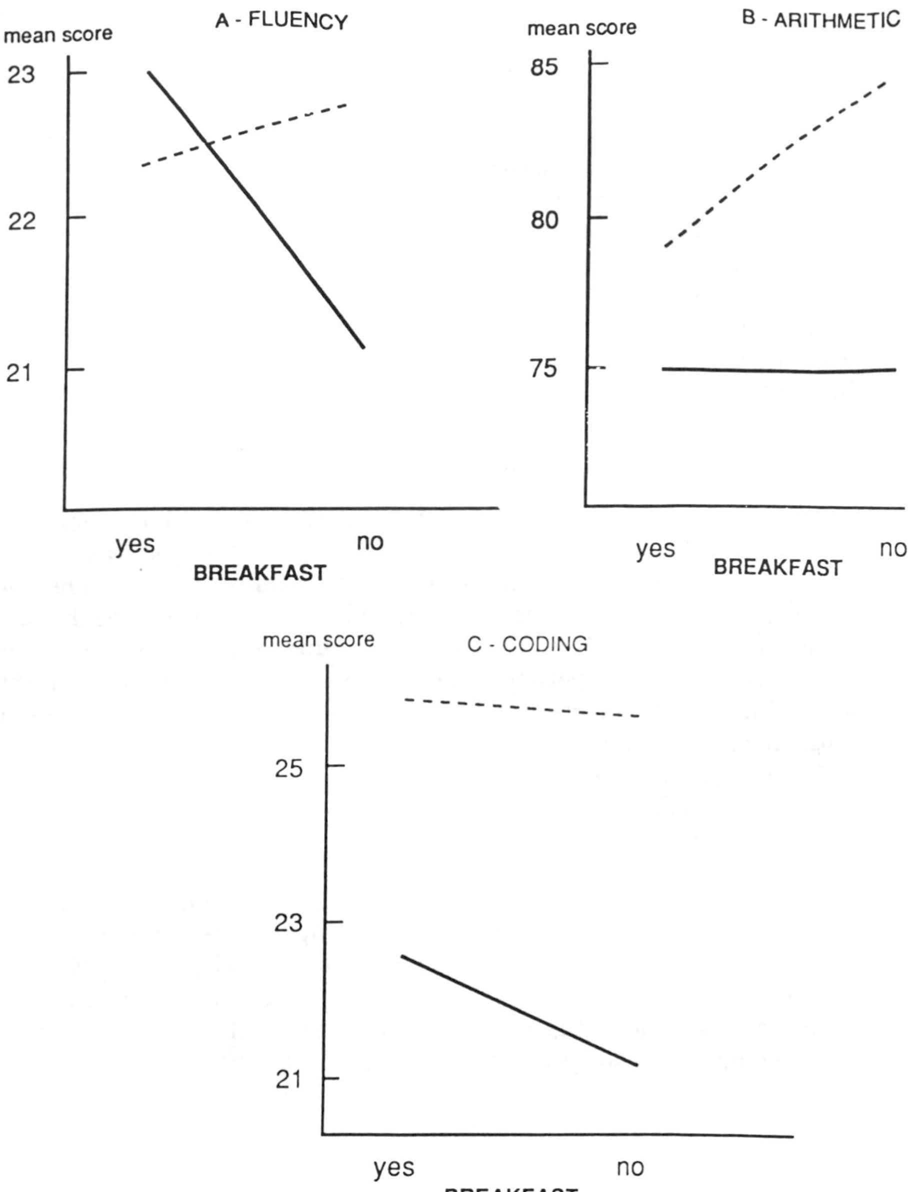

FIGURE 21.2 Influence of prior nutritional status on the relationship between hunger and learning. Mean scores by group in fluency, arithmetic, and coding. ——, combined malnourished group, n = 60; — — — —, control group, n = 30.

trol children . . . missing breakfast could be a serious contributor to poor school achievement in undernourished children. . . . School meals could be targeted to undernourished children."

Although the stated purpose of the school breakfast program is to prevent the consequences of hunger, a second associated benefit is improved attendance. The results of a study of school breakfast program participation in an industrial suburb of Boston showed "improvements in achievement test scores, absence and tardiness" rates of participating as compared with nonparticipating children, with the data evaluation controlled for sex, ethnicity, grade in school and preschool breakfast test scores, and absence and tardiness rates (Myers et al., 1989).

Effect of School Lunch

The study of School Nutrition Programs of 1981 found that overall 24-hour intake of nutrients for consumers of school lunches was higher when compared with the daily intake of children who do not consume school lunch (Radzikowski & Gale, 1984). Differences in growth were found to be small, and, for the most part, nutritional status measurements did not differ between consumers and nonconsumers of the school lunches (Vermeersch et al., 1984). The school lunch and other programs improve dietary intake more than nutritional status.

It is a major concern for the school nurse to keep children enrolled in the school feeding programs. When possible, breakfast programs should be instituted in all schools serving disadvantaged children (e.g., income below 1.85 of the poverty level). In most settings, the school nurse can use her judgment and authority to obtain certification for free lunches on the basis of hardship. For example, the child with a family income at just twice the poverty level is unlikely to be able to afford lunch in school. Confidence must always be maintained so that a poor child living in a community where it is unusual or considered shameful to be poor does not feel singled out for ridicule.

SUMMARY

The school years are formative for a child. Good nutritional habits go along with good habits of all kind. The following guide for the school years is adapted from Dwyer and Freedland (1988) in their description of child health procedures. The school nurse and health service should

1. Monitor nutritional status as an indicator of health and well-being.

2. Provide good examples and guidance to instill healthy habits and attitudes about nutrition.
3. Encourage good food and food programs in the school.
4. Promote physical activity and group participation (as opposed to spectator) sports.
5. Maintain a supportive environment for overweight children. Be sure to encourage physical activity and modest dieting to control weight for these children.
6. Encourage foods with roughage and fiber (rather than sticky sweets) for general and dental health.
7. Educate children to distinguish between valid and bogus food claims. For example, fruit "drinks" are advertised as a good source of vitamin C, but fruit juices are more nutritious.
8. Promote a pattern of foods that are nutritious, culturally acceptable, and affordable.
9. Be sure to address issues of tobacco, alcohol, and illegal drug use early.

ACKNOWLEDGMENTS

The section of this chapter, school-based nutrition education, and a part of the summary were drawn from an unpublished manuscript kindly provided by Christine Olson, PhD, RD, of Cornell University.

The authors thank Melanie MacLennon, MD, for her assistance in the preparation of this chapter.

REFERENCES

American Academy of Pediatrics. (1987). *School health: A guide for health professionals.* Elk Grove Village, IL: American Academy of Pediatrics.

Dwyer, J. T., & Freedland, J. (1968). Nutrition services. In H. M. Wallace, G. Ryan, Jr., & A. C. Ogelsby (Eds.), *Maternal and child health practices* (3rd ed, pp. 261–282). Oakland, CA: Third World.

Kalina, B. B., Philipps, C. A., & Minns, H. V. (1989). The NET program: A ten-year perspective. *J. Nutr. Educ., 21*, 38–42.

Karp, R. J., Haaz, W., Starko, K., & Gorman, J. (1974). Iron deficiency in families of iron deficient inner-city school children. *Am J Dis Child, 128*, 18–20.

Karp, R. J., Nuchpakdee, M., Fairorth, J., & Gorman, J. M. (1976). The school health service as a means of entry into the inner-city family for the identification of malnourished children. *Am J. Clin Nutrition, 29*, 216–218.

Katz, M. S. (1976). *A history of compulsory education laws* (Fastback Series, No. 75). Bicentenial Series.

Kempe, C. H. (1973). A practical approach to the protection of the abused child and rehabilitation of the abusing parent. *Pediatrics, 51*(Suppl.), 804–809.

Myers, A. F., Sampson, A. E., Weitzman, M., et al. (1989). School breakfast and school performance. *Am J Dis Child, 143*, 1234–1239.

Nader, P. R. (1988). School health services. In H. M. Wallace, G. Ryan, Jr., & A. C. Oglesby (Eds.), *Maternal and child health practices* (3rd ed., pp. 463–482). Oakland, CA: Third Party.

Olds, D. L., & Kitzman, H. (1990). Can home visitation improve the health of women and children at environmental risk? *Pediatrics, 86*, 108–116.

Pigg, R. M., Jr. (1989). The contribution of school health programs to the broader goals of public health: The American experience. *J. Sch. Health, 59*, 25–30.

Pollitt, E., Gersovitz, M., & Gargiulo, M. (1978). Educational benefits of the United States school feeding programs: A critical review of the literature. *Am J Pub Health, 68*, 477–481.

Radzikowski, J., & Gale, S. (1984). Requirements for the National Evaluation of School Nutrition Programs. *Am J Clin Nut, 40*(Suppl.), 365–367.

Read, M. (1973). Malnutrition, hunger and behavior: II. Hunger school feeding programs and behavior. *J Am Diet Assoc., 63*, 386–391.

Simeon, D. T., & Grantham-McGregor, S. (1989). Effects of missing breakfast on the cognitive function of school children of differing nutritional status. *Am J Clin Nutrition, 49*, 646–53.

Vermeersch, J., Hanes, S., & Gale, S. (1984). The National Evaluation of School Nutrition Programs: Program impact on anthropometric measures. *Am J Clin Nutr., 40*(Suppl.), 414–424.

22

Clinical Involvement With Children Born to Drug-Addicted Mothers

James Rempel, RN, MS

Given the massive social and biologic pathology of the crack era, the inner-city maternity/newborn unit where I have worked for 10 years as clinical manager has been under siege. It was simultaneously understaffed and overcrowded. Babies were being detoxified, treated for syphilis, ventilated for severe prematurity and respiratory distress, and finally "boarded" as they waited for foster care. We spent our time engaged in crisis intervention that involved chaotic attempts to assess parental competence and extended family support and to determine whether the mother was domiciled with sufficient income to care for the baby.

Given the time needed to treat medical problems and to sort out the varied psychosocial problems, the babies stayed for extended periods in a hospital often ill-equipped to nurture them. Some stayed up to 1 1/2 years while waiting for foster care. Their behavior was highly variable, affected both by the institutional care and the sequelae from intrauterine drug exposure. Some babies shook. Some appeared to have a voracious appetite and then vomited frequently. Approximately 5% to 10% of the babies were irritable enough to require sedation. Certain babies were deceptively normal, but if I watched carefully as they got older, I could see they were depressed and slept excessively. A few actually appeared psychotic. Many were gaze aversive and difficult to engage visually. Certain abnormalities persisted even though some of the children were fortunate enough to spend their early lives in an emotionally safe, boarder baby room where staff was dedicated exclusively to nurturance. It was clear that "hospitalism" was developing right before my eyes (Spitz, 1945).

I have participated in the detoxification of 3,000 drug-exposed newborns. The majority tested positive for cocaine metabolites, but they were probably exposed to multiple toxins rather than isolated alcohol, heroin, or cocaine abuse. Certainly, many mothers gave a history of multiple drug use. So a premature or small for gestational age baby with abnormal neurobehavioral signs probably was exposed to any number of substances such as those listed earlier, as well as sedatives, nicotine, caffeine, and even insecticides that are at times mixed in crack/cocaine.

Most of the mothers had no prenatal care. Many were homeless. Some lived and gave birth in abandoned cars. Many mothers had a history of being physically or sexually abused. Some had cocaine-related psychiatric problems. Too many mothers ate poorly, especially during binges.

Models for drug treatment of narcotics-addicted pregnant women and mothers have demonstrated clearly that comprehensive services delivered prenatally and continued postnatally can radically reduce both morbidity and mortality of the infants. Studies by pioneers in the field, such as Finnegan (1979) in Philadelphia and Brotman et al. (1985) in New York have shown that prenatal and pediatric services delivered within a drug treatment program can increase birth weight and head circumference, and reduce perinatal infections, infant mortality, neglect and abuse among other things. Despite these successes, such programs have not been widely reproduced. This is a very unfortunate response to a desperate need.

SUMMARY

The following guidelines are provided to manage the transition from the inpatient hospital setting to outpatient health care. This is a difficult process given the chaotic nature of the foster care system and the fragility of the mothers and grandmothers caring for the children.

1. Health care must be personalized. The child needs to be discharged to a specific health care facility and not to "the clinic" or "the well-baby station."

2. The facility must provide continuity of care.
3. Easy access is needed to developmental and mental health resources, as well as to specialized AIDS care.
4. Social service support is absolutely essential for families caring for these vulnerable children.
5. Above all, society at large must commit itself to a preventive drug treatment infrastructure oriented to addicted families so that the pathology can be minimized or prevented completely.

REFERENCES

Brotman, R., Hutson, D., & Suffet, F. (1985). *Pregnant addicts and their children.* Valhalla, NY: Center for Comprehensive Health Practice, New York Medical College.

Finnegan, L. (1979). Pathophysiology and behavioral effects of transplacental transfer of narcotic drugs to fetuses and neonates of narcotic dependent women. *Bulletin of Narcotics, 31*, 1–59.

Spitz, R. A. (1945). Hospitalism. *Psychoanalyt Stud Children, 1*, 53–74.

23

At Special Risk: Homeless Children

Ellis Arnstein, MD, Denise Paone, RN, and Andrea Berne, RN

The decade of the 1980s witnessed an enormous increase in the number of homeless people in the United States. The growing number represents the unwanted outcome of a range of public policy decisions, and economic and social pressures that have been created by society at large. For decades there has been a substantial number of homeless adult alcoholics and other substance abusers evident in urban areas, whereas the recent increase in numbers reflects the presence of chronically mentally ill and, for the first time, families with young children.

IMPACT OF HOMELESSNESS ON CHILDREN

For much of the 1980s, families were the fastest-growing group among the homeless. The number of homeless families in New York City remained around 600 (with 1,400 children) through the 1960s and 1970s, whereas by 1982 there were 1,134 families, and by 1987–88 there were approximately 5,200 families including more than 12,000 children (Lopez et al., 1988). These numbers represent only those families known to the city's welfare agency and receiving temporary shelter; there may well have been additional families "residing" in parks, bus stations, subways, and so on. Other urban areas throughout the country experienced similar phenomena, with significant spread to more rural environments as well (Wright & Weber, 1987). Although there is little or no way to assess the numbers accurately, an estimate of 100,000 homeless children was made in 1988 (Institute of Medicine, 1988).

HEALTH AND NUTRITIONAL CONSEQUENCES OF HOMELESSNESS

In keeping with the demographic characteristics of the homeless, most past and present studies looking at health and nutrition among the homeless have focused primarily on the single-adult homeless population. During the past several years (i.e., since 1985), increasing attention has been paid in the medical literature to the health and nutritional status of homeless children and their families, with a wide range of findings. The Table 23.1 summarizes the pertinent findings of these studies and several subsequent ones, along with some comments regarding each. In general, these studies suggest that the degree of impact of homelessness on children's health, nutrition, and developmental status varies directly with the duration of homelessness.

SPECTRUM OF HARM DONE TO CHILDREN

These two cases represent part of the spectrum of harm done to children in the context of homelessness. It is possible to present children with relatively modest nutritional consequences of homelessness.

David

Consider David, a 3-year-old boy who has lived with his mother and two sisters at the Martinique Hotel in New York City for 9 months, and before that, five different "short-stay" hotels over a 6-month period.

His mother, who had received no prenatal care, and, having moved so much, was not receiving formulas and food from WIC. David was switched to whole milk at six months of age. He is a "poor eater," but drinks a lot of milk, 6 to 8 glasses a day. His weight is at the 90th and height at the 50th percentile. An elevated ZPP and a mild anemia suggested either iron deficiency, lead poisoning, or both. His evaluation showed an iron deficiency anemia with a normal lead result. David was placed on iron and given a follow-up appointment in 1 month. Care was entirely within the support system for the hotel-bound families.

TABLE 23.1 Summary of Studies on Health and Nutritional Status of Homeless Children and Their Families

Study	Findings	Comment
Bassuk & Rubin (1987) (see Bassuk, et al., 1986)	82 families, 156 children in Massachusetts shelters; high levels of developmental data, anxiety and depression, and learning disabilities	High rate of parental mental health disorders may have exaggerated impact on these children
Acker, Fierman, & Dreyer (1987)	Children from shelters seen at NYC hospital OPD; high rates of delayed immunization, elevated mean FEP & number of children with controls. Tabulation of heights and weights demonstrated skewing toward 5th-25th percentiles	Findings suggest high risk for nutritional deficiencies, but sample is biased toward those attending clinic
Alperstein, Rappaport, & Flanigan (1988)	Children from shelters seen at NYC hospital OPD; high rates of delayed immunization, elevated blood lead levels	Findings document lack of primary care. No assessment of recent undernutrition included. Also, sample biased towards users of care
Miller & Lin (1988)	82 families, 185 children sheltered in King County, Washington; Self-reported health data: ear infections, asthma, g-i problems, anemia and mental health problems most common. Significant numbers of children were obese (37/105)	Obesity much more prevalent than under-growth: 75% of females over 10 years were obese. Families did use health care visits for well-child care, but nutritional status was not raised as an issue by them
Lewis & Myers (1989)	133 families, 213 children sheltered in Boston area; 85% of children had a regular source of care. 95% had normal developmental screening results (DDST)	No evidence of under-growth or undernutrition, no evidence of developmental delay beyond expected frequency, upon entry into shelter (i.e., newly homeless)

A second story does not have such a happy ending.

Tammy

Tammy moved to the Martinique at 3 weeks of age with her 28-year-old mother. On evaluation at WIC, the nutritionist noticed the baby was wheezing. Mrs. P. said that she had no way to get to Bellevue and "it was too cold and rainy to take her out." The nutritionist told the mother that the "blue medical van" was parked in front of the hotel until 5 p.m. and the mother could take Tammy there, but she did not go that day.

Two weeks later Tammy was brought to the health van at the hotel with a bad diaper rash from moniliasis. Her height and weight were at the 30th percentile. Tammy returned twice that month because the rash had not cleared. By 5 months old Tammy had one hospitilization for bronchiolitis, but her growth and development were normal for age. Several weeks later she came to the van with more wheezing. The monilial infection was obvious. Tammy was not in any acute distress. However, it was noted that her weight had dropped off to the 10th percentile. Two weeks later, she was admitted to the hospital, and a diagnosis of AIDS was made. Initially, the hotel support team and the hospital social worker worked closely with Mrs. P. to arrange for permanent housing so that Tammy could be discharged to the care of her mother. But Mrs. P. stopped visiting the hospital and did not respond to numerous outreach efforts. Finally, after 2 months, Tammy was placed in a special home for children with AIDS.

WHAT MUST BE DONE

As noted in several chapters, there is an inverse correlation between economic and health status. With respect to homelessness, just as governmental policies can exacerbate the problems of those living in poverty, alternative policies and attitudes can have an ameliorating effect.

Regarding the specific nutritional impact of homelessness, some of the recommendations of the Institute of Medicine are worth repeating here: "Because even the most prudent and imaginative parents in homeless families cannot provide adequate nutrition for young children at existing levels of food stamp benefits, such benefits should be recalculated to reflect realistic expenses to meet nutritional requirements. . . . Because many homeless women are pregnant and a growing number of homeless people are children, it is especially important that the WIC Program be strengthened in order to address comprehensively the nutritional needs of pregnant women and young children."

And while these recommendations are valid for all families in poverty, including the homeless, they become particularly important for families who remain homeless for an extended period, when the secondary impact of homelessness becomes marked.

REFERENCES

Acker, P. J., Fierman, A. H., & Dreyer, B. P. (1987). An assessment of parameters of health care and nutrition in homeless children [abstract]. *American J. Dis. Children, 141*, 388.

Alperstein, G., Rappaport, C., & Flanigan, J. M. (1988). Health problems of homeless children in New York City. *Am. J. Public Health, 78*, 1232–1233.

Bassuk, E., & Rubin, L. (1987). Homeless children: A neglected population. *American Journal of Orthopsychiatry, 57*, 279–286.

Bassuk, E. L., Rubin, L., & Lauriat, A. S. (1986). Characteristics of sheltered homeless families. *American J. Public Health, 76*, 1097–1101.

Brickner, P. W., Scanlan, B. C., Brennan, B., et al. (1986). Homeless persons and health care. *Annals of Internal Medicine, 104*, 405–409.

Institute of Medicine, Committee on Health Care for Homeless People. (1988). *Institute of Medicine: Homelessness, health, and human needs*. Washington, DC: National Academy Press.

Lewis, M. R., & Meyers, A. F. (1989). The growth and development status of homeless children entering shelters in Boston. *Pub. Health Reports, 104*, 247- .

Lopez, K., Salamone, M, & Tobier, N. (1988). *Health service delivery systems within HRA's adult and family shelters*. New York: Adult Services Agency of the New York City Human Resources Administration.

Miller, D. S., & Lin, E. H. B. (1988). Children in sheltered homeless families: Reported health status and use of health services. *Pediatrics, 81*, 668–673.

Sprowal, C. (1986, November). Unpublished data presented at the Public Health Interest Consortium for New York City.

Wright, J. D., & Weber, E. (1987). *Homelessness and health*. New York: McGraw-Hill

24

Nutrition Policy: Children in Poverty

Marion Nestle, PhD, MPH

Whether or not experts consider the United States to have a national policy for children and their families, they conclude that present policies are inadequate. For example, Republican members of the Select Committee on Children (1990) write, "National policy is rooted in the Constitutions and laws of the Federal and state governments, the functions of more than 83,000 units of governments and the myriad of judicial decisions. . . . So the real problem is a conflict among competing policies, not the absence of policy."

This conclusion derives from the rising socioeconomic gap between rich and poor families, the increasing proportion of children in poverty, and the declining international rank in infant mortality rates observed in this country.

Nutrition is only one component of U.S. governmental policies for children, but it is a highly visible index of their effectiveness. That current nutrition policies are also inadequate is documented by increasing reports of hunger and demands for federal food and income assistance among women and children, institutionalization of private-sector soup kitchens and food pantries established to meet unmet needs (Cohen & Burt, 1989), and findings of insufficient or inappropriate food intake, mild to moderate malnutrition, obesity, and impaired growth, health, and social behavior among low-income children (Kotch & Shackelford, 1989).

This chapter reviews the history of federal food and nutrition policies for low-income children and their families, describes the principal programs that presently constitute these policies, and suggests ways in which these policies might be restructured to improve their ability to meet immediate as well as long-term nutritional needs.

HISTORICAL BACKGROUND

The earliest child nutrition programs in the United States began just a century ago when public concern about children in the labor force, recent advances in medicine, and the development of state and local health departments created an environment favorable to social action for child welfare. The first child nutrition program appeared in 1893 when private centers were established in New York City to distribute uncontaminated milk to children and to teach mothers about healthy feeding practices. Five years later, the city's Bureau of Child Hygiene took over these activities and became the first governmental agency to assume responsibility for the health of children (Schmidt, 1973).

Federal Role in Nutrition Services

Federal involvement in child nutrition began in 1909 when participants at the first White House Conference on Children recommended that a federal Children's Bureau be created (see Table 24.1). From its inception in 1912, the Children's Bureau campaigned for comprehensive health and nutrition services for children and families through studies, publications, conferences, grants, and legislation.

Further White House Conferences were convened once each decade from 1919 to 1970. Over the years, these Conferences called for policies that would establish adequate nutrition as a fundamental right of children, increase access of disadvantaged children to health and nutrition services, expand and improve food programs, and promote nutrition education in the schools.

Policy demands of the 1919 Conference led Congress to pass the 1921 Maternity and Infancy (Sheppard-Towner) Act. This unprecedented and highly controversial legislation established federal responsibility for maternal and child health (MCH) through grants to state health agencies. Because services were to be made available to all residents—including those of racial minorities—the act was denounced by the American Medical Association and by Congress as an "imported

TABLE 24.1. Selected Federal Initiatives to Improve the Diet and Nutritional Status of Children.

1909	First White House Conference on Children emphasizes importance of comprehensive health services for children and recommends creation of a Children's Bureau.
1912	Children's Bureau established to investigate and report on matters pertaining to the welfare of children.
1914	Children's Bureau recommends nutrition as component of prenatal care.
1919	Second White House Conference on Children proposes legislation to provide health services to mothers and infants.
1921	Maternity and Infancy (Sheppard-Towner) Act provides grants to states to develop health and nutrition services.
1929	Maternity and Infancy Act repealed in response to concerns that it reflects socialist philosophy.
1933	Amendments to the Agricultural Act permit purchase of surplus commodities for donation to child nutrition and school lunch programs.
1935	Social Security Act of 1935 passed. Title V of this act again authorizes grants to states for health and nutrition services to mothers and children.
1941	First *Recommended Dietary Allowances* sets standards for nutrient intake of infants and children.
1946	National School Lunch Program established.
1954	Special Milk Program established.
1963-67	Amendments to Social Security Act expand health and nutrition services for low-income infants.
1965	Title XIX of the Social Security Act authorizes Medicaid.
1966	Child Nutrition Act passed. School Breakfast Program established.
1967	Early and Periodic Screening, Diagnosis, and Treatment (EPSDT) program established under Medicaid.
1968	Senate Select Committee on Nutrition and Human Needs created; sets child nutrition as major priority for action.
1968-70	Ten-State and Preschool Nutrition Surveys and *Hunger, U.S.A* report evidence of malnutrition among children in poverty.
1969	White House Conference on Food, Nutrition, and Health calls for programs to prevent childhood malnutrition.
1972	WIC authorized.
1977	Food and Agricultural Act and Child Nutrition and National School Lunch Amendments passed.
1979	DHEW issues *Healthy People: The Surgeon General's Report on Health Promotion and Disease Prevention* with goals for improved child health.
1980	DHHS issues *Promoting Health/Preventing Disease: Objectives for the Nation* with specific goals for improvement of child nutrition. The Surgeon General's Workshop on Maternal and Infant Health recommends policies to improve nutritional status.
1981	Select Panel for the Promotion of Child Health submits *Better Health for Our Children:A National Strategy* with nutrition recommendations.

Continued

TABLE 24.1. ***Continued.***

1988	DHHS publishes *Surgeon General's Report on Nutrition and Health* with policy recommendations for child nutrition.
1990	Year 2000 National health promotion objectives identify maternal and child health and nutrition as priorities for preventive services.

Sources: Egan, 1977; National Commission, 1988; Schmidt, 1973; U.S. Department of Health, 1988, 1990.

socialistic scheme," and it was repealed in 1929 (Schmidt, 1973). Within the next 5 years, more than half the states reduced or eliminated MCH services.

As the need for services grew during the depressed economy of the 1930s, Congress reinstated many of the provisions of the Sheppard-Towner Act by passing the Social Security Act of 1935. Title V of this act authorized federal grants to states for a variety of health and nutrition services. Amendments in the 1960s established special MCH projects as well as Medicaid, the principal source of funding for health and nutrition services for low-income families. Further amendments in 1981 established the Maternal and Child Health Block grant, which allocated funding for virtually all MCH services to the states.

This transfer of responsibility reflected a federal philosophy that favored decentralized administration of individual health and welfare programs and weakened the ability of the Children's Bureau to promote comprehensive services. During the 1960s, the bureau was reorganized repeatedly, and its multiple health and welfare functions were divided and transferred to other agencies. Remnants of the bureau remain today in the Department of Health and Human Services (DHHS) Bureau of Maternal and Child Health, which oversees federal administration of Title V Block Grant funds.

Federal Food Assistance Programs

In the 1930s, widespread unemployment, poverty, and hunger in the midst of an oversupply of many farm products stimulated Congress to create programs to distribute surplus agricultural commodities as food relief. Amendments to the Agricultural Act of 1933 authorized donation of surplus foods to child nutrition and school lunch programs; these programs were organized more formally in 1935 (Kerr, 1988). During the next 20 years, Congress established the School Lunch, School Breakfast, Special Milk, and Food Stamp Programs.

In the late 1960s, national surveys and private inquiries reported evidence of malnutrition among children in selected poverty areas. These findings shocked the nation and stimulated Congress to expand eligibility and benefits for existing programs and to establish WIC. From 1969 to 1977, annual federal expenditures for food assistance increased from $1 to $8 billion and exceeded $20 billion in 1988 (Matsumoto, 1989).

CURRENT FOOD AND NUTRITION PROGRAMS

A recent inventory describes more than 125 federal programs designed at least in part to aid children and their families through income support, social services, education and training, health care, and housing—as well as nutrition (Select Committee on Children, 1990). Virtually all of these programs affect the nutritional status of low-income children either directly or indirectly. Of these programs, 23 are targeted specifically to children of low or limited income; another 34 emphasize benefits to such children. Total expenditures for these 57 programs were estimated to be $132 billion in 1986.

Table 24.2 summarizes the major features of the principal federal programs designed wholly or in part to improve the nutritional status of low-income children and their families through food assistance, nutrition education, nutrition services, or income assistance.

Food Assistance

Federal food assistance programs provide meals and snacks, foods, or vouchers to purchase food. Four programs—Child Care Food, National School Lunch, School Breakfast, and Summer Food Service—provide meals to children in day care, school, camp, or other institutional settings. Three—Commodity Assistance, Commodity Supplemental Food, and Special Milk—provide free or subsidized milk or other food commodities to children enrolled in (or, in some cases, excluded from) other food assistance programs (Select Committee on Children, 1990).

The two most important food assistance programs—Food Stamps and WIC—reach children through their caretakers. Food Stamps entitle individuals and families to buy coupons that can be used as cash to purchase food for home consumption. WIC provides specific foods or vouchers for foods for infants and young children who have been determined to be at risk because of inadequate nutrition or income.

All of these programs are administered at the federal level by the USDA through its Food and Nutrition Service. Funding is distributed to local agencies through the states. Most are entitlements; anyone

TABLE 24.2 Principal Federal Programs Designed at Least in Part to Improve the Nutritional Status of Low-Income Children Through Food Assistance, Services, Education, or Income

Program	Target Group	Federal/State/Local Administration	Entitlement Status	1989 (or 1990 Estimated) Funding (in $ millions)	1988 Participants (millions)	Type of Benefit
Food Assistance						
Child Care Food	Preschool children in child care	USDA/states/agencies	Yes	669	1.3	Free or subsidized meals and snacks
Commodity Assistance	Children enrolled in School Lunch, Child Care Food, and Summer Food programs	USDA/states/schools and agencies	Yes	530		Commodity support for lunch and breakfast programs
Commodity Supplemental Food	Infants and children not enrolled in WIC	USDA/states/agencies	No	60	0.131 in 18 states and D.C.	Free commodities
Food Stamps	Individuals and families	USDA/state and local welfare departments	Yes	10,300 (82% to households with children)	18.8 (51% children under 18)	Coupons to purchase food for home use
National School Lunch	School age children	USDA/states/schools	Yes	3,100	24.2 (60% of eligible)	Free or subsidized lunches
School Breakfast	School age children	USDA/states/schools	Yes	510	3.69	Free or subsidized breakfasts
Special Milk	Preschool and school age children in nonprofit agencies' programs	USDA/states/agencies	Yes	21	1.0	Free or subsidized milk
Special Supplemental Food Program for Women, Infants, and Children (WIC)	Infants and children through age 4 determined to be at nutritional risk	USDA/states/agencies	No	1,900	3.6 (31% infants, 47% children)	Food or vouchers for food, education, access to health care
Summer Food Service	School age children in summer programs, camps	USDA/states/agencies	Yes	149	1.6	Free meals
Temporary Emergency Food Assistance (TEFAP)	Households, emergency food distribution sites	USDA/states/agencies	No	(170)	15	Free commodities

Nutrition Education						
Expanded Food and Nutrition Education (EFNEP)	Families and youth	USDA Extension/states/ land-grant colleges	No	(58)		Outreach by para-professionals
Nutrition Education and Training (NET)	Teachers and food service personnel	USDA/states/schools	No	(5)	2.2	Instructional materials and training
Nutrition Services						
Community Food and Nutrition (CFN)	Communities	DHHS Office of Community Services/states/community agencies	No	2	22 communities	Grants for anti-hunger projects
Community Health Centers	Medically underserved	DHHS Health Resources and Services Admin./regions/agencies	No	415	5.4 (one-third are children)	Nutrition screening, referral, treatment
Head Start	Preschool children	DHHS Office of human Development Services/states/agencies	No	1,200	0.448	Nutrition assessment, education, meals, snacks
Maternal and Child Health Services Block Grant	Young children with limited access to health services	DHHS Health Resources and Services Admin/states/agencies	No	554		Nutrition screening, counseling, education, referral; SPRANS* *grants.*
Medicaid—Early and Periodic Screening, Diagnosis, and Treatment (EPSDT)	Eligible children	DHHS Health Care Financing Admin./states	Yes	6 (for all Medicaid benefits to children)	10 (all programs for children)	Nutrition screening, referral, treatment
Income Assistance						
Aid to Families with Dependent Children (AFDC)	Children of absent, deceased, disabled and unemployed parents	DHHS Office of Family Assistance, Family Support Administration/ states/county welfare offices	Yes	9,000 benefits 1,500 admin.	10.9 (7.3 children)	Cash payments

*Special Projects of Regional and National Significance to expand and improve nutrition services for mothers and children.

Sources: Community Nutrition Institute, 1990; FRAC, 1989; Kalina et al., 1989; Matsumoto, 1989; Randall et al., 1989; Select *Committee on* Children, 1990.

who meets eligibility criteria is guaranteed the right to receive benefits. The one notable exception is WIC; current estimates suggest that only about half of eligible individuals receive benefits.

Since the late 1970s, overall expenditures for USDA programs have more than doubled, and the number of participants in some—though not all—child nutrition programs has increased. From the dollar figures in Table 24.2, it appears that about 75% of the $20 billion expenditure is targeted at children. Because benefits may overlap, the number of children reached by these programs is difficult to estimate. If 27 million—daily participants in the National School Lunch program plus infants and children enrolled in WIC—can be assumed to be a minimum, the average food assistance benefit in 1989 just exceeded $550 per child.

Nutrition Education

The WIC program and all the nutrition service programs listed in Table 24.2 provide nutrition training or materials to parents, teachers, agency staff members, or the children themselves. Two programs specifically target low-income children and their families. EFNEP, through active outreach efforts, trains volunteers from low-income communities to teach community members about ways to improve dietary intake.

The Nutrition Education and Training Program (NET) uses the school lunch and other child nutrition programs as laboratories to teach principles of healthy diets to teachers, food service and other school staff, and children from preschool through 12 grades (Kalina et al., 1989). NET is designed to reach all children in participating schools, regardless of family income. Although originally funded in 1978 for $26 million, its budget was reduced to $5 million in 1982 and has remained at that level ever since.

Nutrition Services

At least five programs administered by DHHS mandate nutrition services—assessment, counseling, referral, or treatment—usually as relatively minor components of more comprehensive health programs for low-income children and families. In recent years, DHHS has expanded Medicaid eligibility (Hays, 1990); initiated demonstration projects to test the efficacy of case-managed, comprehensive health, and nutrition services; authorized grants for Special Projects of Regional and National Significance to improve such services; initiated a surveillance system to track pediatric malnutrition; and reported on efforts to monitor the nutritional status of the low-income population.

Income Assistance

Although not directly a nutrition program, Aid to Families with Dependent Children (AFDC) is the principal source of federal financial assistance to children up to age 18 or 19 whose low-income parents are deceased, disabled, continually absent from the home, or unemployed. Eligibility for AFDC provides automatic eligibility for many health and nutrition programs. States establish levels of financial need and benefit but in nearly all cases maximum benefit levels fall below 100% of need (Children's Defense Fund, 1990a). In 1989, $9 billion in AFDC benefits was distributed to 10.9 million recipients, of which 7.3 million were children (Select Committee on Children, 1990). This calculates to an average annual benefit of $825 per person.

NUTRITION PROGRAMS: ISSUES OF CONCERN

Taken together, federal nutrition programs were expected to constitute a "safety net" for low-income families. Yet within the past 10 years, surveys conducted by more than 200 church, community, advocacy, and governmental groups have reported hunger and inadequate access to food among the poor, especially toward the end of the month, and especially among women and children, at least in part because federal funding does not meet needs (Cohen & Burt, 1989).

Inadequate Benefits

In 1989, monthly AFDC benefits for a family of three ranged from a low of 15% of the federal poverty level in Alabama to a high of 88% in California and exceeded 50% of the poverty level in only 21 states. The combined benefits from AFDC and Food Stamps reached the poverty level in only two states (Alaska and California). The average Food Stamp benefit was $0.54 per meal (Children's Defense Fund, 1990a). The lower the income, the higher proportion spent on food; low-income families spend 30% or more of their income on food, an amount that exceeds the average Food Stamp allotment by at least 10%.

Declining Benefits

From the early to the mid–1980s, the value of AFDC benefits declined by 18.5% for a family of four. The Food Stamp budget fell, in real terms, by 35% (Select Committee on Children, 1989), and funding for child nutrition programs (excluding WIC) declined by 29% (Children's Defense Fund, 1988). The president's 1991 budget proposals for food assistance include increases only for WIC and Temporary Emergency Food Assistance Program (TEFAP); reductions proposed for child nutrition programs total a 9% decline from the previous year (Children's Defense Fund, 1990b).

Declining Participation

From 1979 to 1986, the proportion of children in poverty who received AFDC benefits declined from 72% to 60%. About 50% of eligible women and children are unable to obtain WIC benefits, and the Food Stamp program fails to reach about a third of those who are eligible. Food Stamp participation fell from 1980 to 1986, despite a growth of 3 million in the population below the poverty line, and 2.1 million eligible children were dropped from the National School Lunch Program (Children's Defense Fund, 1988).

Increased Administrative Complexity and Cost

Analyses by groups across the entire political spectrum have documented barriers to participation in health and welfare programs raised by the multiplicity of responsible agencies, separate authorizing legislation, inconsistencies in eligibility requirements, and complexity of regulations. As shown in Table 24.2, the programs are administered by separate agencies with separate missions, constituents, and budgets. Such complexity makes access difficult. (Table 24.3 suggests how to refer patients to appropriate programs). It is also costly; although administrative costs are not specified for most programs, they include $1.5 of the 10.5 billion allocated for AFDC. For at least some programs, much of the administrative work is devoted to prevention of fraud.

Program Accomplishments

Although it seems evident that feeding hungry children should improve their health and nutritional status, it has proved difficult for researchers to attribute such benefits directly to food assistance programs. Potential differences between participants and nonparticipants complicate research as do unrelated changes in health and nutritional status that may occur over time. Controlling for just the principal variables requires large numbers of study subjects and is very expensive.

TABLE 24.3. Access to Federal Food and Nutrition Programs for Low-Income Children and Families.

Because responsibility for food and income assistance programs is fragmented among many agencies and because cities vary in the ways they implement these programs, it is helpful to know how to refer patients to programs for which they may be eligible.

For information about:	Write or telephone:
Food Stamps and AFDC (Aid to Families with Dependent Children)	City welfare (human resources, social services) offices
School Breakfast School Lunch Head Start	School district
WIC (Special Supplemental Food Program for Women, Infants and Children)	Health department
EFNEP (Expanded Food and Nutrition Education Program)	Cooperative extension
Referral to local food and welfare programs	Public library, reference desk
Referral to local food advocacy groups	Food Research and Action Center 1875 Connecticut Ave. N.W., Suite 540 Washington, DC 20009—202-986-2200
Federal data on poverty among women and children	Center on Budget and Policy Priorities 777 North Capitol Street, N.E. Washington, DC 20002—202-408-1080
MCH advocacy	Children's Defense Fund 25 E. St., N.W. Washington, DC 20001—202-628-8787
Federal MCH programs	Select Committee on Children, Youth, and Families, U.S. House of Representatives Ford Building, Room 385 Washington, DC 20515—202-226-7660

Nevertheless, some evidence suggests the value of nutrition programs independent of other factors. Researchers have associated NET and EFNEP with improved dietary knowledge, attitudes, and behavior (Kalina et al., 1989; Randall et al., 1989); the School Breakfast Program with improved scores on standardized achievement tests (Meyers et al., 1989); and Food Stamps with improved nutritional status (Allen & Gadson, 1984). WIC has been researched most thoroughly. From 1974 to 1985, at least 30 studies examined its impact but were only able to demonstrate small improvements on low and mean birth weight. In response to a mandate by Congress, the USDA sponsored a comprehensive evaluation of the program. This study identified small but positive benefits of program participation on infant birth weight and head circumference, dietary intake, and improved cognitive development, especially among children at highest risk (Rush et al., 1988).

POLICY OPTIONS FOR THE UNITED STATES

The methods for development of effective health, nutrition, and welfare programs for low-income children that were proposed early in this century remain valid. They invariably include three basic components: access to prenatal and pediatric care, coordination of Maternal and Child Health (MCH) services, and provision of comprehensive services that meet the full range of health and welfare needs of children and their families.

The value of these recommendations is demonstrated by previous experience in the United States and also by the experience of other developed nations, especially those in Western Europe. Although European countries have not entirely eliminated child poverty, they have assigned a higher national priority to child welfare and their problems are not as severe. For all children, regardless of income, these countries provide access to health care, eligibility for assistance, and day care and schools where meals are served; they do not require means testing (verification of low-income status) for program eligibility, and they do not limit benefits to a restricted proportion of eligible children (Miller, 1990).

Despite these lessons, current U.S. federal policy recommendations do not sufficiently promote the three elements of successful MCH strategies. The principal process for development of national health policy is the creation of successive 10-year plans to attain specific goals and objectives in defined areas of health promotion and disease prevention. In 1980, in the first of these plans, one of the MCH objectives called for participation by virtually all infants in a system of primary health care that includes nutrition services. This objective has not yet been achieved (Office of Maternal and Child Health, 1988).

The Public Health Service recently released a new set of objectives to be achieved by the year 2000 (U.S. Department of Health, 1990). Among these objectives are several that address service and protection: (a) to increase to at least 90% the proportion of pregnant women and infants who receive risk-appropriate care; (b) to increase the proportion of infants who receive recommended primary care services to at least 90%; and (c) to increase the proportion of low-income people who have received appropriate screening, immunization, and counseling services to 50% for adults, to 90% of infants up to 24 months, and to 80% of children ages 2 to 12. Unless there are immediate improvements in administrative and funding priorities for child health, nutrition, and welfare programs, even these limited goals are unlikely to be achieved by the year 2000.

Many agencies and groups have recommended changes in present federal nutrition policies to increase the availability of food and income assistance to poor families. These recommendations call for increased funding for food assistance programs, expansion of participation eligibility, conversion of programs (especially WIC) to entitlements, and elimination of administrative barriers (Cohen & Burt, 1989; FRAC, 1989; Select Committee on Children, 1989). These are critical, short-term measures for alleviation of program inadequacies, and they deserve support.

More important, however, is the broader, longer-term need for a system that guarantees children the right to adequate nutrition, education, health, and welfare services, regardless of income. The key elements of such a system necessarily include

- Employment for parents and caretakers
- Access to health care services
- Housing
- Day care (with meals)
- Schools (with meals)

To approach this ideal is not impossible. Countries with far fewer resources have succeeded in instituting policies that promote many of these elements. In this country, the institution of such policies will require some basic restructuring of attitudes and priorities, and a major shift in the distribution of national expenditures.

SUMMARY

That the future of this nation rests with its children is self-evident. That successful citizens must be healthy, well educated, and decently sheltered and fed also seems self-evident, yet present U.S. policies do not adequately promote these basic human rights. Throughout the developed world, nations establish the welfare of children as a national priority through universal health care, free and compulsory education, and a social welfare system available to all. If the United States is to retain its position of world leadership, our government must develop similar policies that promote the health, nutrition, and welfare of all children. When it does, malnutrition among American children in poverty will become an issue of concern only to historians.

Acknowledgments

The author thanks Sally Guttmacher, Jill Kagan, Lorraine Klerman, and Lynn Parker for providing many of the documents on which this analysis is based.

REFERENCES

Allen, J., & Gadson, K. (1984). Food consumption and nutritional status of low-income households. *National Food Rev, 26*, 27–31.

Children's Defense Fund. (1988). *A children's defense budget FY 1989*. Washington, DC: Children's Defense Fund.

Children's Defense Fund. (1990a). *S.O.S. America! A children's defense budget*. Washington, DC: Children's Defense Fund.

Children's Defense Fund. (1990b). *The nation's investment in children: An analysis of the president's FY 1991 budget proposals*. Washington, DC: Children's Defense Fund.

Cohen, B. E., & Burt, M. R. (1989, October). Eliminating hunger: Food security policy for the 1990s. Washington, DC: The Urban Institute.

Community Nutrition Institute. (1990). Food, nutrition budget: Spending analysis 1991. *NI Weekly Rep* Feb. *1*, 4–6.

Egan, M. C. (1977). Federal nutrition support programs for children. *Pediatr Clin North Am, 24*, 229–239.

FRAC. (1989, March). *Fact sheets on the federal food programs*. Washington, DC: Food Research and Action Center.

Hays, L. B. (1990). From the Health Care Financing Administration. *JAMA, 263*, 496.

Kalina, B. B., Phillipps, C. A., & Minns, H. V. (1989). The NET program: A ten-year perspective. *J Nutr Educ, 21*, 38–42.

Kerr, N. A. (1988). The evolution of USDA surplus disposal programs. *National Food Rev, 11* (3), 25–30.

Kotch, J., & Shackelford, J. (1989, June). *The nutritional status of low-income preschool children in the United States: A review of the literature*. Washington, DC: Food Research and Action Center.

Matsumoto, M. (1989, October-December). Recent trends in domestic food programs. *National Food Rev, 12* (4), 34–36.

Meyers, A. F., Sampson, A. E., Weitzman, M., et al. (1989). School breakfast program and school performance. *Am J Dis Children, 143*, 1234–1239.

Miller, C. A. (1990, March 20). *Child health: Lessons from developed nations* (Testimony before the Select Committee on Children, Youth, and Families). Washington, DC: U.S. House of Representatives.

National Commission to Prevent Infant Mortality. (1988). *A historic day for children: Program supplement.* Washington, DC.

Office of Maternal and Child Health. (1988). Progress toward achieving the 1990 objectives for pregnancy and infant health. *JAMA, 2660*, 770–771.

Randall, M. J., Brink, M. S., & Joy, A. B. (1989). EFNEP: An investment in America's future. *J Nutr Educ, 21*, 276–279.

Rush, D. (1988). The National WIC Evaluation: Evaluation of the Special Supplemental Food Program for Women, Infants, and Children. *Am J Clin Nutr, 48*(Suppl.), 389–519.

Schmidt, W. M. (1973). The development of health services for mothers and children in the United States. *Am J Public Health, 63*, 419–427.

Select Committee on Children, Youth, and Families. (1989). *Children and families: Key trends in the 1980s* (Staff Report, December 1988). Washington DC: U.S. House of Representatives.

Select Committee on Children, Youth, and Families. (1990, February 27). *Federal programs affecting children and their families, 1990: A report together with additional minority views.* Washington, DC: U.S. House of Representatives.

U.S. Department of Health and Human Services. (1980). *Promoting health/preventing disease: Objectives for the nation.* Washington, DC: U.S. Government Printing Office.

U.S. Department of Health and Human Services. (1988). The Surgeon General's Report on Nutrition and Health. Washington, DC: U.S. Government Printing Office.

U.S. Department of Health and Human Services. (1990). *Healthy people 2000: National health promotion and disease prevention objectives* (Conference Edition). Washington, DC: U.S. Government Printing Office.

25

Paralyses of Response

David M. Rosen, PhD, JD

As is amply demonstrated in this text, poverty creates malnutrition and malnutrition can radically inhibit the life chances of the child. There would seem to be a theoretically simple and elegant solution to this problem; provide the poor with more money or food. Indeed, some of the most successful antipoverty programs, such as WIC, follow this model. They give poor people what they need.

Yet despite the demonstrated success of such programs, there is significant political and professional resistance to the idea of solving the problem of poverty through direct transfers of economic resources to the poor. Such an approach subverts key cultural and ideological tenets of American society namely that economic reward should flow from individual effort. Consequently, antipoverty programs are invariably laden with ambiguity; they seek not to eliminate poverty directly but to create some minimum conditions that will allow the poor themselves to escape from poverty.

We have been unwilling to admit that the American Dream has been permanently denied to some individuals or communities based on race, ethnicity, or social class status. "Poverty," we have said, "exists in 'pockets,' not in the heartland." This long-held view of American society is challenged by the spector of a permanent underclass. There is a growing conviction that for many Americans the American Dream will be permanently denied and that those who are born poor will probably die poor. Indeed, in 1987 over five million children under the age of six lived below the federal poverty line (*Five Million Children*, 1990).

A virtual corollary to this approach is the analysis of those behaviors among the poor that purportedly serve to enhance or inhibit the escape from poverty (Lewis, 1966; Wilson, 1987). Though it is recognized that the poor have behavioral characteristics that are distinctive, the concept of a "culture of poverty" is an inappropriate and overdetermined concept stemming from a naive sense of the idea of culture (Geertz, 1973; Valentine, 1968).

In fact, the poor are not dysfunctional operators in a limited resource base but are highly adaptive actors in an essentially dysfunctional economic system (Liebow, 1967; Stack, 1974). Poverty creates a powerful environment that shapes people's responses to social situations (see chapter 2). We have the ability, through public policy and personal initiative, to change the environment in which people live.

This is by no means the first time Americans have been forced to confront the issue of poverty in our society. After an abortive "War on Poverty" in the 1960s and early 1970s, poverty in the 1980s and 1990s is occurring under profoundly different circumstances than before. The politics of scarcity and the bogeyman of new taxes have effectively shut down the institutions designed to ameliorate the problems of the very poor. Our leaders seem incapable of distinguishing between a public policy and a public plea. In the 1988 presidential campaign, George Bush's "a thousand points of light" was substituted for "Meals on Wheels" as if to say "Let Them Eat Light."

If the culture of the poor is not defective, the real issues facing the poor are primarily structural and individual. Thus responses need to address the economic and social constraints—the "structures of opportunity"—within which the poor adapt and cope. Moreover, it is necessary to treat the poor as real individuals not as caricatures of a defective culture. Both approaches require the investment of human and monetary resources. The first calls for jobs, industry, and investment, and the second calls for nonbureaucratic individually tailored programs designed to treat poor persons with respect (Schorr & Schorr, 1985). The fact that answers to the problems of poverty may be politically unacceptable should not cause us to turn to politically acceptable formulas that provide no real solutions.

REFERENCES

(1990). *Five million children: A statistical profile of our poorest young children.* New York: National Center for the Study of Children in Poverty, School of Public Health, Columbia University.

Geertz, C. (1973). *The interpretation of culture: Selected essays.* New York: Basic Books.

Liebow, E. (1967). *Tally's corner: A study of negro streetcorner men*. Boston: Little, Brown.

Lewis, O. (1966). The culture of poverty. *Sci Am, 215*, 19–25.

Schorr, D., & Schorr, L. B. (1985). *Within our reach*. New York: Anchor/Doubleday.

Stack, C. (1974). *All our kin: Strategies for survival in a black community*. New York: Harper & Row.

Valentine, C. A. (1968). *Culture of poverty: Critique and counter-proposals*. Chicago: University of Chicago Press.

Wilson, W. J. (1987). *The truly disadvantaged: The underclass and the inner-city*. Chicago: University of Chicago Press.

26

Breaking the Cycle of Poverty

Robert J. Karp, MD

Undernutrition is not an isolated event in the life of an affected preschool and early school age child. Their families are economically dependent and disrupted by marital discord. Single parenthood is common. There is inadequate use of the medical, social, and educational resources available. Other family members are undernourished. The community itself is impoverished.

Moreover, the child's health is often affected by pica, lead poisoning, and increased occurrence of infectious illness. Reduced somatic growth reflects the concomitant effects of iron and possibly zinc deficiency, and inadequate caloric intake. Exposure to toxic substance in utero (specifically alcohol and drugs) may have occurred. Delayed entry into school and poor attendance are likely. The concomitant poor performance may reflect any of the variables noted including the cumulative effects of parental behaviors surrounding the nurturing of the child.

The prevalence of undernutrition in young children and the consequences are related so closely to chronic poverty that one can only rarely distinguish the consequences of these disorders from the consequence of living in the milieu in which undernutrition occurs. This conundrum is more apparent than real and should not paralyze efforts to develop appropriate remedies.

CONSIDER YOUR OPTIONS

No single person or institution has all of the skills or resources necessary to care for the larger social and psychological problems of the disadvantaged. The problem of malnutrition, as one example, is often a symptom as well as a consequence of disadvantage and poverty. Thus, it is best treated by an interdisciplinary team including physician, nurse, nutritionist, social worker, home health worker, and others from outside the medical community such as planners of agriculture, economists, sociologists, and educators (Jellife, 1966; American Academy of Pediatrics, 1992).

But having a team of committed individuals in place can only partly address problems of malnutrition and disadvantage in our society. It is necessary to specify the commitments society as a whole must make to break the cycle of poverty. Without public responsibility for the disadvantaged, all the poor will receive is lip service. "Structures of opportunity" must be provided within which the poor can adapt to the society at large (Schorr, 1990).

PROVIDE SERVICE FOR PEOPLE AND PEOPLE FOR SERVICE

Among industrial democratic societies, we stand out, not for our accomplishments, which are many, or for our wealth, which is great, but for our failures. In the United States, there is a lack both of adequate health insurance and adequate public facilities to serve the poor (Relman, 1989; Woolhandler et al., 1989). These are barriers to health care. Without health insurance, the disadvantaged cannot use the private system for health care. For the most disadvantaged children, services required will be found in the underfunded public sector if they are to be found at all. Moreover, support for the worst off in society begins, as all industrial democracies have realized, with a broad base of support for every one (Williams & Miller, 1992). Otherwise, notes Chamberlin, "for every family whose functioning is improved by some kind of intensive intervention, several more medium-risk families will take their place as their life circumstances change" (Chamberlin, 1992).

But personal commitment is needed to make public policy work. Often, the first step for a person to leave the world of disadvantage is a personal contact with another human being who offers help when it is needed and wanted. It was that one person "in the right place at the right time," who cared enough to listen and to respond who made the difference. Committed people being at "the right place" to establish and maintain trust is a prerequisite for care of the disadvantaged.

RECOGNIZE RISK FACTORS IN THE COMMUNITY

Problems in the community associated with malnutrition include (a) a high prevalence of low-birth-weight infants, single parents, and teen mothers. These require preventive and therapeutic programs for health, parenting, and birth control. Other concerns include (b) the condition of the housing stock. Think of lead poisoning. (c) Is there an excess number of taverns and liquor stores? Think of fetal alcohol effects. (d) Is there an excess number of children in classes for mentally retarded or learning disabled? Think of micronutrient deficiencies, growth retardation, lead poisoning, alcohol exposure, a need for parenting classes, and special Head Start programs for children. (e) Are there adequate facilities for children to play outside? Think of obesity. (f) Are there adequate programs for nutritional supplementation? Is there screening for health and nutrition problems at the local school? Do the schools care about the meals they serve and provide nutritious food and a supportive environment? A health care provider's concern for these problems will draw him or her together with others inside and out of the community to advocate needed changes and guide those changes so that they are effective.

RECOGNIZE THE EARLY SIGNS OF MALNUTRITION

Plans for treatment should be comprehensive because malnutrition is not an isolated occurrence in the lives of affected children. Iron deficiency and growth retardation, for example, have meaning beyond nutrition. Often other family members are malnourished, and the malnutrition may be a signal that other social or medical problems exist in the family. Built into the health care given to a child is the recognition that an abnormal test for hematological status requires more than a prescription for iron and a bit of dietary advice. The diet history should be taken carefully with an ear for the limitations in intake forced by poverty and the food culture of chronic poverty. Each member of a health care team knows of the special risks for this child and each—the dietitian, the nurse, and the social worker—has a role to play in the care of the child.

ADDRESS SOCIAL POLICY ISSUES

In the first chapter of the text, Johnston and Markowitz described the characteristics of developing countries including their inability to respond to social dislocation and malnutrition. By contrast, all industrial democracies, other than the United States, have social policies that take advantage of the wealth generated by free-market economies to maintain the general well-being—including good nutrition—of their people.

The best marker for health of populations is the neonatal mortality (death of infants before 30 days of age per 1,000 live births). Eighteen countries have neonatal mortality rates below our rate of 10.0/1,000 (Wegner, 1988) including all of Scandinavia, Western Europe, and Japan. This raises the question: In what direction is our society going?

The results of policies that nurture and nourish children include remarkable improvements in health and social stability. V. W. Greene, a microbiologist, has observed that great pride is taken by the medical profession in curing the diarrheal disease of individual children, but there is little sense of accomplishment in the medical community when diarrheal disease is prevented. It is not recognized that ignoring the cause for diarrhea, mostly a failure to provide clean water but also a failure to provide nutritious food, is as immoral as ignoring an individual dying child (1984). No person could walk past a hungry child without offering food and still maintain his or her self-respect, but we accept the reality of living in a society that leaves a substantial number of children without adequate support for nutrition and health.

As a youth, the Indian economist, A. Sen, witnessed the great Bengal famine of 1943 when 3 million people died (Sen, 1981). Yet, even at the height of the famine, there was food available, and the starvation was not general. An unskilled and landless work force had been displaced by an economy that was focused on the British war effort. No provision was made for them to work or to eat. Sen maintains that starvation, and by extension malnutrition, occurs when food is considered an entitlement that can be taken from groups of people who are deemed insufficiently valuable to society for them to eat well. At present, vulnerable groups in developing countries and in the United States (e.g., the homeless, teen mothers, and infants of the poor) cannot assert an ownership right to an adequate diet. This is an ugly trend that must be reversed. Greene and Sen are not writing about clean water or preventing famine per se; they are describing the consequences of not considering the responsibilities of an individual member of society to the society in which he or she lives (Sen, 1990).

The origins of the cycle of poverty have no simple or single explanation, nor is there a single path out of the cycle. But as Schorr notes

(1990), nonbureaucratic individually tailored programs designed to treat poor persons with respect are effective. Solutions are "within our reach." If society and the individual can produce the cycle of poverty, then society and the individual can succeed in terminating it. "By comprehensive and efficient Maternal and Child Health Service," writes Cicely Williams, "we can minimize the wretchedness of unwanted and neglected babies, and we can practically abolish the malnutrition due to misuse of foods" (1973).

The case studies in this book were selected from real life, and just as in real life, the outcome of choosing one course of action or another is not entirely predictable. The mothers presented were not chosen because they were heroic figures, but they are good mothers for their children. They are, like all human beings, capable of making choices, and they make them to the best of their abilities. The most difficult task in planning care for patients is to continue to seek trust and commitment in the face of great disappointment.

REFERENCES

American Academy of Pediatrics. (1992). The medical home. Ad Hoc Task Force on Definition of the Medical Home. *Pediatrics, 90*, 774.

Chamberlin, R. W. (1992). Preventing low birthweight, child abuse, and school failure: The need for comprehensive, community wide approaches. *Pediatrics in Rev., 13*, 64–71.

Greene, V. (1984). *Cleanliness and the health revolution.* New York: The Soap and Detergent Association.

Jelliffe, D. B. (1966). *The assessment of nutritional status in the community* (World Health Organization Monograph Series, No. 55, pp. 75, 227, 236). Geneva, Switzerland: World Health Organization.

Relman, A. (1989). Universal health insurance: Its time has come. *NEJM, 320*, 117, 314.

Schorr, L. B. (1990). *Within our reach: Breaking the cycle of disadvantage.* New York: Anchor Press/Doubleday.

Sen, A. (1981). *Poverty and famine.* New York: Oxford University Press.

Sen, A. (1990). Individual freedom as a social commitment. *New York Review of Books, 37*, 49–54.

Wegner, M. (1988). Annual summary of vital statistics—1987. *Pediatrics, 82*, 817–834.

Williams, C. D. (1973). Nutrition and population. *Nut Revs, 31*, 372.

Williams, B. C., & Miller, C. A. (1992). Preventive health care for young children: Findings from a 10-country study and directions for United States policy. *Pediatrics, 89*, 983–998.

Woolhandler, S., Himmelstein, et al. (1989). National health program for the United States: A physician's program. *NEJM, 320*, 107.

Epilogue

Laurence Finberg, MD

This book adds to the literature on childhood nutrition by placing emphasis on the close links between economic distress and poor nutritional practices. When one goes to examine the causes of childhood undernutrition, one invariably finds an extremely complex set of issues related to poverty. Poverty and feeding interact to produce a cascade of events frequently disastrous to the infant and child. In this brief summary I shall target three issues—two related to poverty, one to affluence.

First, in the developing world, the scarcity of adequate energy and protein are complicated by an unsanitary water supply, poor hygiene, and consequent recurrent infection. Popularization of a scientifically based oral rehydration therapy has been enormously helpful in the recovery from single episodes of dehydrating enteric infection. Although there are differences of opinion as to how these solutions should be administered and constituted, there is no question that they are useful. Unfortunately, recovery from a single episode does not assure survival through infancy. Many infants have multiple infections, each episode adding a period of undernutrition. Some of the outcomes still include death, stunting of growth, and cognitive impairment. Thus, although we can estimate the number of times oral hydration therapy corrects dehydration or prevents it, we still do not know what impact this modality has on the overall outcome for poverty-stricken children in the developing world.

Second, in industrial societies, adequate energy and even adequate protein are generally present. However, poor housing and poor parenting skills often associated with poverty and ignorance frequently lead to bad outcomes that could be prevented by assuring safe housing, reducing the likelihood of accidents, and preventing inappropriate dietary practices. Lead poisoning, iron deficiency, and even mild rickets, all of them easily preventable, continue to be seen in the inner cities of the affluent United States. Preventing these interrelated problems will probably result in savings to the economy in the long run.

A final concern for consideration is somewhat new to pediatric nutrition, that is, the subject of the prevention of the degenerative diseases of later life by appropriate nutrition in childhood. One example is the attempt to prevent coronary artery disease. It is now clear that cholesterol levels at the point where there is arterial damage have some influence on the occurrence of coronary occlusion. It is also clear that fatty streaks appear in the aortas of children on high-fat diets by the age of 10 or so. Such lesions, however, are not seen in coronary arteries until much later. What is not clear is whether dietary control in childhood will influence what happens in later life, except in those unusual families where there is a genetic defect producing hypercholesterolemia.

For the general population it certainly seems sensible to eat a diet containing less fat than the current average American diet. In particular, the saturated fat component should be lower than is current, and most agree that 10% of calories should be the upper limit for this dietary constituent. There is also general agreement that 30% of calories as fat is satisfactory for providing energy while not promoting a high cholesterol level.

Thus there is general agreement on advising a "prudent diet" for all Americans, adults and children (older than approximately 2 years of age). There remain differences of opinion on the importance of monitoring cholesterol levels in all children. Part of the reason lies in the fact that this measurement is a very crude surrogate for what one really wants to know. The other part of the objection is that having measured cholesterol, it is not clear (except in the families with genetic defect) that anything beyond the already recommended diet is of any value. In another decade, and perhaps sooner, our tools will be better and our course of action more clearly delineated.

Index